Aleksej Thorevskij

Emergency conditions in oncology

Aleksej Thorevskij

Emergency conditions in oncology

Emergency conditions in patients with malignant tumors and intensive care

ScienciaScripts

Imprint

Any brand names and product names mentioned in this book are subject to trademark, brand or patent protection and are trademarks or registered trademarks of their respective holders. The use of brand names, product names, common names, trade names, product descriptions etc. even without a particular marking in this work is in no way to be construed to mean that such names may be regarded as unrestricted in respect of trademark and brand protection legislation and could thus be used by anyone.

Cover image: www.ingimage.com

This book is a translation from the original published under ISBN 978-620-6-14303-1.

Publisher:
Sciencia Scripts
is a trademark of
Dodo Books Indian Ocean Ltd. and OmniScriptum S.R.L publishing group

120 High Road, East Finchley, London, N2 9ED, United Kingdom
Str. Armeneasca 28/1, office 1, Chisinau MD-2012, Republic of Moldova, Europe
Printed at: see last page
ISBN: 978-620-5-77946-0

Emergency conditions in oncology

Alexei Valentinovich Tkhorevsky

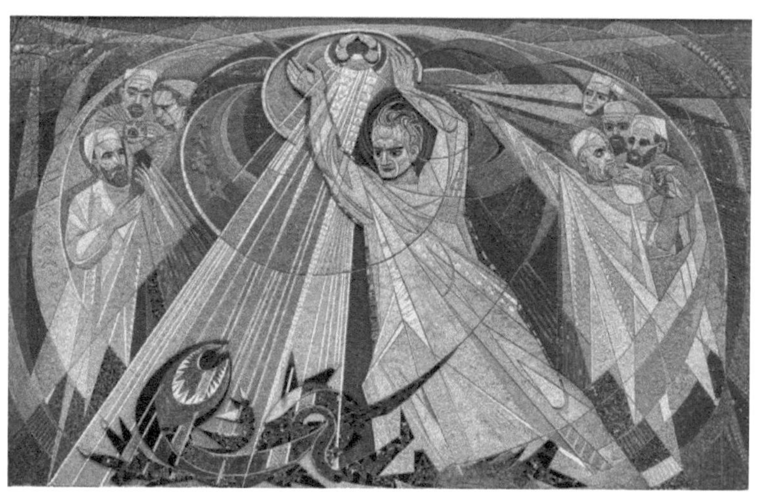

Victory - Galina Zubchenko, Grygoryi Pryshedko (National Sapseur Institute, Kyiv)

INTRODUCTION

Cancer is often seen as a slow and prolonged disease, with insidious onset of symptoms and signs. However, clinical conditions often arise that require urgent evaluation and treatment. Surgical treatment leads to improved survival and reduced morbidity. Most oncologic emergencies occur early in the disease process and are related to the severity of the tumor process or the effects of chemotherapy drugs, but some may arise later in the treatment process or even at relapse. Patients may have other comorbidities such as coronary artery disease, stroke, or hyperglycemia that may not be related to cancer. Cancer patients should always be evaluated in the same way as patients without the disease. A comprehensive clinical evaluation of each patient will help identify problems early.

This book reviews medical conditions specific to patients with malignant tumors. The clinical protocols of the European Society for Medical Oncology (ESMO) and other current protocols for the treatment and prevention of emergency conditions in cancer patients are displayed. Each chapter is accompanied by a recommended reading list. Examples of clinical problems with a step-by-step algorithm are reviewed.

The book will be useful to all physicians who nobly treat this ailment. The author expresses his sincere gratitude to the founders and management of the Academician Yuri Prokopovich Spizhenko Medical Center "Spizhenko Clinic", within whose walls this work was performed, my friends from the National Cancer Institute, my superiors (who always emphasized that there are no "little things" in intensive care), my family, friends and colleagues (who helped me be strong and confident in myself).

The material was translated and collected by Alexey Valentinovich Tkhorevsky, associate professor at the Department of Anesthesiology, UVMA.

CONTENTS

CHAPTER 1. EFFECTS OF CANCER PROCESSES ON ORGANS AND SYSTEMS

Central nervous system

Altered mental status.

Altered mental status is the most common central nervous system (CNS) manifestation in cancer patients in the intensive care unit (ICU). Common differential diagnoses are discussed below. If they can be ruled out and the patient has not received excessive sedation or narcotic analgesics, sepsis should be ruled out in the patient. Altered mental status is a reliable, although nonspecific, sign of sepsis, which is accompanied by a high mortality rate among cancer patients.

1. *Intracranial volumetric lesions*

A history of headache, nausea, vomiting, or seizures combined with cerebral edema and other signs. Elevated intracranial pressure suggests intracranial vascular damage. A moderate increase in intracranial pressure by itself is relatively well tolerated, but when the intracranial pressure becomes critical, the brain matter will shift in the direction of least resistance, leading to the formation of an intercerebral bulge through the dura mater or *foramen magnum.*

2. *Primary CNS tumors*

They are manifested by focal neurological signs, depending on from localization.

3. *Secondary (metastatic) tumors*

Approximately 15-30% of secondary tumors are accompanied by first-onset seizures. Common malignancies associated with metastases to the brain include breast, lung, kidney, and melanoma.

4. *Cerebral hemorrhage*

Cerebral hemorrhage is associated with acute promyelocytic leukemia as a direct complication of brain metastases or associated thrombocytopenia.

5. *Subdural hematoma*

Acute subdural hematomas are accompanied by fluctuations in the level of consciousness and hemiparesis.

6. *Brain abscess*

Brain abscess accounts for 30% of CNS infections in cancer patients.

a) Clinically evident increased intracranial pressure and neurological deficits are late signs.

(b) Usually presents with fever, headache, drowsiness, confusion, and seizures.

c) Usually seen in patients with leukemia or head and neck tumors.

Other reasons for changes in mental status in critically ill patients cancer patients

Leptomeningeal metastases

a) May show signs of increased intracranial pressure and hydrocephalus.

(b) Acute leukemia, lymphoma, and breast cancer, as well as carcinomas of the central nervous system, are frequent causes.

2. Cerebrovascular accident (CVA). Often occurs in cancer patients. As in all patients, CVC may be thrombotic, hemorrhagic, or embolic in nature.

a) Most patients have focal neurological signs and headaches.

(b) Seizures are common, especially in hemorrhagic disorders of cerebral circulation.

c) Embolic CPV in cancer patients may be associated with septic emboli, especially in patients with fungal infections (e.g., aspergillosis).

Metabolic encephalopathies. Lethargy, weakness, somnolence, coma, agitation or psychosis, focal or generalized seizures can all result from metabolic disorders. Absence of focal neurological signs is indicative of metabolic encephalopathy.

Examples include:

(a) Hypercalcemia

(b) hyponatremia

(c) hypomagnesemia

(d) hypoglycemia

(e) Uraemia

(f) Hyperglycemia (e.g., hyperosmolar non-ketotic acidosis)

(g) Wernicke's encephalopathy

h) Disorders of porphyrin metabolism

4. *Convulsive seizures/postictal state.* A postictal state is often seen after a seizure with a generalized onset; it is characterized by deep sleep, headaches, confusion and muscle pain and lasts from a few minutes to several hours. Occasionally, Todd's palsy (transient neurological deficits, usually weakness, in the limb opposite the focus of pathological electrical activity) may be detected during this period. In patients with primary and secondary tumors (especially hemispheric ones), seizures are observed in most cases.

(a) Differential diagnosis excludes CVC, CNS infection, brain injury or drug withdrawal, and central nervous system cancer as causes of seizures.

(b) Signs of tongue biting, loss of bladder/intestinal control, and plantar flexion reflexes may be found in the immediate postictal period.

(c) The presence of lateralized focal signs suggests that seizures may have a focal origin.

(d) Prolonged coma after a generalized seizure or transient hemiparesis (Todd's palsy) after a Jacksonian, focal or generalized seizure is more common in patients with seizures secondary to a focal lesion than in those with seizures resulting from other diseases.

5. *Cerebral leukostasis*

In patients with hyperleukocytosis (defined as a peripheral blood white blood cell count >100,000/mm3), white blood cell clots can cause cerebral vessel occlusion, and the clinic may manifest as blurred vision, dizziness, ataxia, stupor or coma or intracranial hemorrhage.

a) Hemorrhage occurs as a result of leukostatic occlusion arterioles and capillaries with endothelial cell damage, capillary leakage and destruction of small vessels.

(b) Retinal hemorrhages are indicative of Cancer: central nervous system with intracranial hemorrhages, so a thorough examination should be done frequently.

6. Increased viscosity syndrome (EPS)

Excessive increase in serum paraprotein levels or pronounced leukocytosis can lead to increased serum viscosity, sedimentation, and decreased perfusion of the microcirculation with stasis. Can affect any organ system; however, the characteristic clinical manifestations are seen in the lungs and CNS.

a) Patients may have visual disturbances or loss of vision.

(b) Characteristic retinopathy is present with venous dilation (with "sausage link" or "wagon" segmentation), microaneurysms, hemorrhages, exudate, and sometimes edema.

c) Similar vascular changes can be observed in the bulbar zone of the conjunctiva.

(d) Other clinical manifestations may include headache, dizziness, Jacksonian and generalized seizures, drowsiness, lethargy, coma, and auditory disturbances, including hearing loss.

7. *CNS infections*

Patients with cancer are susceptible to various CNS infections, including meningitis, brain abscess, and encephalitis.

(a) Meningitis is most common in patients with impaired cell-mediated immunity and is usually caused by Cryptococcus neoformans or Listeria monocytogenes.

(b) Patients with meningitis have fever, headache, and altered mental status.

(c) All cancer patients with fever and altered mental status should undergo a lumbar puncture, preceded by

computed tomography (CT) scan of the head (if there is suspicion of lesions of the meninges).

d) Encephalitis is most commonly caused by herpes viruses (simplex or zoster) or Toxoplasma gondii.

(e) Patients with encephalitis usually present with signs of meningeal irritation (fever, headache, neck stiffness) and signs of altered mental status. Confusion may progress to stupor and coma; focal neurological signs and seizures are common.

Spinal cord compression. Significant spinal cord compression occurs as a result of epidural metastases and is most commonly seen in breast, lung, or prostate cancer with spreading disease.

As a rule, the main complaint is back pain (90% of patients), which may be accompanied by weakness, autonomic dysfunction, sensory disturbances, ataxia and flexion reflexes. The neurological deficit is determined by the level of the spinal cord involved.

1. Compression by metastasis usually arises from three places:

(a) Spinal column (85%)

(b) paravertebral spaces (10-15%)

c) epidural space (rare)

2. The distribution along the spine is approximately as follows:

(a) Thoracic (60-70%)

(b) Lumbar (20-30%)

(c) Cervical (10%)

Central Nervous System: Diagnostic Assessment in the Intensive Care Unit.

1. history, physical examination and careful neurological evaluation, signs of lateral displacement, ocular fundus examination, and signs of increased intracranial pressure.

2. *laboratory tests must include*:

(a) Arterial blood gases

(b) Electrolytes and serum glucose

(c) Calcium, magnesium, and phosphorus

(d) Renal and liver function tests

e) determination of serum viscosity, especially in cases of multiple myeloma or other paraprotein-producing tumors

3. *Computed tomography*

Computed tomography of the head is the diagnostic test of choice for detecting mass lesions, midline displacement, intracranial hemorrhage, or hydrocephalus.

4. *Magnetic resonance imaging (MRI)*

MRI is a sensitive test for detecting intracerebral metastases and to differentiate between vascular and tumor masses. It is also the study of choice for evaluation of intramedullary, intradural, and extramedullary spinal lesions.

5. *Myelography*

Myelography provides an indirect image of the spinal cord and nerve roots from the foramen magnum to the sacrum. It is the "gold standard" in assessing spinal cord involvement by a tumor. It is especially useful for patients with contraindications to MRI (e.g., orthopedic patients) and patients who are scheduled for radiosurgery or radiation therapy.

6. Lumbar puncture (LP). LP is most useful for diagnosing meningeal carcinomatosis, CNS leukemia, and CNS infections.

Central Nervous System: Acute Therapy in the Intensive Care Unit.

1. Increased intracranial pressure with dislocation

a) Glucocorticoid therapy will improve neurological deficits in 70% of patients with symptomatic brain metastases by reducing vasogenic brain edema.

An initial dose of 10 mg dexamethasone may be given intravenously, followed by 16 mg per day in three or four divided doses in the most appropriate way.

Patients who do not respond to the standard dose may improve when the dose is increased to 100 mg/day.

(b) Osmotherapy using agents such as urea or mannitol is used to rapidly reduce intracranial pressure in patients with known or suspected intracranial metastases. Mannitol 1.5-2.0 g/kg as a 20% solution may be administered by slow intravenous (IV) infusion. The total dose should not exceed 120 g/day. If co-administered with furosemide may further enhance the effects of mannitol, but is also associated with the risk of dehydration and hypokalemia.

(c) Hyperventilation may be administered in patients who show signs of cerebral dislocation. They should be promptly intubated and ventilated to maintain arterial PCO_2 at 25-30 mmHg.

However, the use of this method is controversial. Some authors believe that the favorable effect of hyperventilation lasts only 6 h. To date, there is no conclusive evidence that this therapeutic intervention changes the outcome in these patients.

(d) Consultation with a neurosurgeon is necessary for the vast majority of patients.

2. Seizures

a) Position the patient sideways to prevent aspiration and protect the airway.

(b) Correct any metabolic changes or hypoxemia.

(c) If the seizure is prolonged, acute control is achieved with lorazepam (Ativan) 1-10 mg intravenously, or a continuous infusion may be used. Alternatively, diazepam (Valium™) 5-10 mg intravenously may be repeated at 5-10 min intervals up to 30 mg.

Another useful drug to quickly stop seizures is the intravenous administration of propofol (Diprivan™) by an anesthesiologist.

(d) Long-term seizure control can usually be established with intravenous phenytoin (Dilantin™). The loading dose is 15 mg/kg intravenously (50 mg/min). Fosphenytoin may also be used.

(e) Intracerebral metastases should be treated with corticosteroids, chemotherapy, radiation, or surgery depending on the specific lesion.

3. Spinal cord compression

Providing palliative care is considered reasonable.

(a) Radiotherapy and surgical decompression are the cornerstones of treatment.

(b) Chemotherapy with nitrogen mustard or cyclophosphamide has been used effectively, usually in combination with radiation, to treat spinal cord compression caused by lymphoma or Hodgkin's disease.

4. Other methods of treatment

a) Leukophoresis is one of the therapy options for severe symptomatic leukocytosis with leukostasis.

(b) If hydrocephalus is present, it should be treated by emergency relief and bypass.

(c) Radiotherapy is currently the most commonly used treatment for palliation of cerebral metastases.

5. General supportive therapy

a) Stress ulcer prophylaxis in the form of antacids, sucralfate, or H2-receptor antagonists.

b) Prevention of deep venous thrombosis (DVT) should include, unless contraindicated, the use of subcutaneous heparin (or low molecular weight heparin) and/or the use of sequential compression techniques.

(c) Nutritional support should be provided to replenish malnourished patients and to maintain good nutrition in patients at risk of malnutrition due to cancer or its sequelae.

d) Appropriate antimicrobial therapy.

e) Foley catheterization for urinary retention, prophylaxis constipation caused by immobility and autonomic dysfunction.

Textbook of Critical Care, 8th Edition Editors : Jean-Louis Vincent & Frederick A. Moore & Rinaldo Bellomo & John J. Marini.

Pulmonary complications.

The lungs are often involved in cancer patients, with 75-90% of pulmonary complications are secondary to infection. Noninfectious complications include those caused by chemotherapy (e.g., bleomycin), chest irradiation, and lung resection. Respiratory failure in cancer patients requiring mechanical ventilation is associated with 75% mortality.

Pulmonary infiltrates. In patients with systemic cancer, the differential diagnosis of pulmonary infiltrates visible on a normal chest x-ray is extensive.

1. Localized infiltrates confined to a single lobe or segment in a patient with a compatible history most often represent a bacterial process.

2. Diffuse bilateral infiltrates most often indicate opportunistic infection caused by treated lung injury, or lymphogenic spread of carcinoma.

3. Bilateral perihilar (cortical) infiltrates in patients who gain weight rapidly confirm the diagnosis of fluid overload.

4. Pulmonary infiltrates after bone marrow transplantation.

a) Life-threatening infections usually occur within the first 100 days after transplantation.

b) During the first 30 days after transplantation, the most common pathogens for pneumonia are bacteria or fungi.

(c) Interstitial pneumonia (diffuse non-bacterial pneumonia) is the predominant problem after transplantation with a syndrome consisting of dyspnea, unproductive cough, hypoxemia, and diffuse bilateral infiltrates occurring within 30-100 days after transplantation.

(d) Cytomegalovirus (CMV) pneumonia accounts for the majority of interstitial pneumonitis. The prevalence of CMV infection appears to be related to loss of immunity during pre-transplant irradiation and the development of graft-recipient disease.

(e) Obliterating bronchiolitis syndrome as a manifestation of graft disease.

(f) Pulmonary hypertension.

g) Diffuse alveolar hemorrhage caused by infectious and non-infectious causes.

5. *Diagnosis.*

a) Chest radiographs are never diagnostic for any one disease.

(b) Sputum cultures and special stains of tracheobronchial secretions (KOH, India ink) should be performed routinely. Colonization of the upper respiratory tract as well as inadequate sputum secretion may make identification of the pathogen(s) difficult.

c) Blood cultures for fungal and bacterial organisms.

d) Viral titers (especially CMV).

e) Daily determination of serum lactate levels can have

some value in patients with respiratory failure with RDSV.

Elevated serum lactate levels may precede deterioration of arterial blood gas indices and development of diffuse infiltrates

(f) Bronchoscopy with bronchoalveolar lavage (BAL) has a diagnostic sensitivity of 80-90% and is the procedure of choice in cancer patients with diffuse infiltrates.

1. BAL is most useful for diagnosing opportunistic infections (e.g., Pneumocystis carinii (jirovecii), viruses such as CMV, fungi, and mycobacteria).

2 This procedure is also useful for diagnosing intraparenchymatous pulmonary hemorrhage.

3. BAL is safe for patients with thrombocytopenia and mechanical ventilation who cannot tolerate transbronchial biopsy.

g) Open lung biopsy should be performed only in patients with comorbidities, discomfort and financial difficulties.

6. *Treatment.*

a) Early empirical use of broad-spectrum antibiotics.

(b) In patients in whom fever persists despite the use of antibiotics, amphotericin B and liposomal amphotericin have been shown to reduce mortality from infection.

(c) Ganciclovir and hyperimmune globulin have been shown to improve survival in patients with interstitial pneumonia.

Pulmonary leukostasis. Leukostasis with obstruction of blood flow in small pulmonary vessels, is a consequence of intravascular accumulation of immature, rigid myeloblasts, observed mainly in acute myelogenous leukemia (AML) and chronic myelogenous leukemia (CML) patients in the blast phase.

Stasis and vascular distension lead to local hypoxia. Release of intracellular enzymes and procoagulants leads to vascular and pulmonary parenchyma damage.

1. Signs and Symptoms: Progressive shortness of breath and/or change in mental status.

2. Diagnosis

a) White blood cell count is usually >150,000/mm^3 .

(b) Arterial blood gases. True hypoxemia develops as a result of impaired pulmonary gas exchange. False low PaO values$_2$ can occur because a large number of blasts consume oxygen in the blood sample itself. The longer the interval between sampling and analysis, the lower the measured PaO$_2$. This can make it difficult to assess gas exchange.

(c) Pulse oximetry may be useful to monitor the adequacy of arterial oxygen saturation.

(d) A chest X-ray may be normal or show diffuse nodular infiltrates.

3. treatment

(a) Myeloblast counts >50,000/mm^3 require immediate treatment to reduce the total white blood cell count to 20-60% within hours of syndrome recognition.

(b) Leukopheresis.

(c) Chemotherapy (e.g., daunorubicin, cytosine-arabinoside, hydroxyurea).

d) Adequate hydration.

e) Prophylaxis of urate nephropathy should be started with allopurinol and urine alkalinization.

f) Hemodynamic monitoring is recommended.

g) If ARDS occurs as a result of leukostasis, the following should be performed promptly:

1. Fluid restoration of blood volume.

2. Cardiac output and hemodynamics should be optimized by increasing inotropic agents as needed.

3. Pulmonary vasoconstriction should be treated with a combination of volume augmentation, inotropic agents, and supplemental O_2 .

4. Mechanical ventilation should be performed when necessary to achieve normal pH, pCO_2 and PO_2 >60 with acceptable FiO_2 .

5. Consideration of a provision (pronunciation)

Treatment-induced lung injury

1. lung injury caused by chemotherapy. A large number of chemotherapeutic agents can cause pulmonary toxicity, either actively or delayed years after therapy. Commonly used agents with known pulmonary toxicity include alkylating agents (e.g., cyclophosphamide, carmustine, chlorambucil, melphalan, busulfan), antimetabolites (e.g., methotrexate, azathioprine), anticancer antibiotics (e.g., bleomycin, mitomycin), and alkaloids (e.g., vincristine). Pulmonary toxicity can take the following forms:

(a) Non-cardiogenic pulmonary edema (NPCI)

(b) Chronic pneumonitis and fibrosis

(c) Hypersensitivity pneumonitis (e.g., procarbazine, methotrexate, bleomycin)

2. Radiation-induced pulmonary toxicity

Radiation pneumonitis is a clinical syndrome of shortness of breath, cough, and fever that develops in conjunction with fuzzy, cloudy pulmonary infiltrates that may progress to dense alveolar consolidation after treatment with ionizing radiation.

(a) The likelihood of developing radiation-induced lung damage depends on a number of variables, including total dose, dose fractionation, volume of lung exposed, and prior irradiation and chemotherapy

(b) Pathophysiology.

1. Direct effect of ionizing particles on alveolar structure.

2. Generation of high-energy oxygen-free radicals in amounts exceeding those of normal enzymatic systems (peroxidase, superoxide dismutase).

3. Release of vasoactive substances such as histamine and bradykinin, which affect capillary permeability and pulmonary vascular resistance. The resulting lung damage may be greater than the exposed area.

(c) 5% to 15% of patients develop radiation pneumonitis.

d) Symptoms may appear 1-6 months after completion of chest irradiation.

Cardiovascular system

Cardiac tamponade. Cardiac tamponade is a life-threatening condition caused by increased intrapericardial pressure, which leads to restriction of ventricular diastolic filling and decreased stroke volume and cardiac output.

1. Disseminated etiology in cancer patients

a) Metastatic pericardial tumors.

1. Much more often lead to tamponade than primary pericardial tumors.

2. Tamponade is caused either by the formation of an effusion or by squeezing.

3. Lung and breast cancer, lymphoma, leukemia, and melanoma account for 80% of the metastatic causes of cardiac tamponade.

(b) Primary pericardial tumors

c) Postradial pericarditis with fibrosis. The pericardium is the most frequent site of radiation damage. The period between radiation therapy and the onset of clinical pericardial disease can be years.

(d) The tumor surrounds the heart.

2. *Clinical manifestations*

(a) Symptoms are often nonspecific, but usually include a feeling of fullness in the chest, pain in the pericardium or interscapular region, restlessness, shortness of breath, and orthopnea.

(b) Clinical signs include altered mental status, hypotension, tachycardia, pulse pressure in narrow arteries, distant heart tones with attenuated apical pulse, tachypnea, palpitations, oliguria, and diaphoresis (excessive sweating).

Other attributes include the following:

1. Pulsus paradoxus

2. Evart's sign (area of blunting under the angle of the left scapula)

3. Cussmaul's sign (neck veins swell on inhalation)

3. *Diagnosis*

a) Clinical suspicion: The key to recognizing tamponade is to consider two diagnoses.

(b) Chest radiography.

1. A large globular shadow of the heart ("water bottle"). If the pericardial fluid volume is <250 ml, the cardiac silhouette may be normal.

2. The lung fields are usually clear.

3. Pleural effusions are frequent accompanying findings.

c) Electrocardiogram (ECG).

1. Sinus tachycardia.

2. Low QRS voltage (<5 mV).

3. Electrical oscillations that result from the heart contracting in a filled pericardial sac. The alternating QRS complexes are most specific for pericardial effusion.

(d) Echocardiography allows rapid and definitive diagnosis of tamponade. Two-dimensional echocardiography is more sensitive than M-mode. Results include the following:

1. Prolonged diastolic collapse or inversion of the free wall of the right atrium.

2. Early diastolic collapse of the free wall of the right ventricle.

3. Effusions up to 30 ml in size are detected early on echocardiography (seen as echonegative space).

e) Pulmonary artery catheterization (Swan-Ganz).

1. Elevation of pulmonary capillary pressure in the right atrium with a marked decrease on the x-axis and no significant decrease on the y-axis ("square root sign").

2. Decreased cardiac output, stroke volume, systemic arterial pressure and mixed venous blood oxygen saturation (SvO2).

3. Alignment of all diastolic pressure readings

(f) MRI is also diagnostic, but it is expensive and time-consuming compared to echocardiography.

(g) Diagnostic pericardiocentesis.

1. Cytology to detect the presence of malignant cells

2. Gram staining and smear for acid-fast bacilli, culture and sensitivity, cell count and differential analysis.

3. Protein and lactic dehydrogenase (LDH) content

4. therapy

a) Therapeutic pericardiocentesis should be performed immediately in hemodynamically compromised patients.

1. Two-dimensional echocardiography-guided pericardiocentesis is successful in 95% of cases without serious complications.

2. Reaccumulation of fluid can occur in malignant effusions, but can be prevented by chemical sclerosing (e.g., tetracycline), radiation therapy, or surgery (e.g., tetracycline). or surgery (e.g., pleuropericardial window or pericardectomy).

Myocardial tissue damage

1. Disseminated etiology in cancer patients

a) Anthracycline antibiotics (e.g., doxorubicin and daunorubicin).

(b) Mitoxantrone: Total dose >100-140 mg/m^2 may cause congestive heart failure and worsen pre-existing anthracycline cardiomyopathy.

(c) Cyclophosphamide: Doses >100-120 mg/kg over 2 days may lead to congestive heart failure and hemorrhagic myocarditis/pericarditis and necrosis.

(d) Busulfan: A normal oral daily dose may cause endocardial fibrosis.

e) Interferons: In normal doses, interferons can aggravate underlying heart disease.

(f) Mitomycin C: Standard doses may cause myocardial damage.

(g) Radiation-induced cardiomyopathy causes dose-dependent endocardial and myocardial fibrosis, which can lead to restrictive cardiomyopathy.

2. Diagnostics

(a) Endomyocardial biopsy: valuable for establishing the etiology of cardiac lesions in patients who may have received chemotherapy and for detecting subclinical cardiac lesions. Anthracyclines cause characteristic degenerative changes in myocytes.

(b) Blood pool scan with ECG to accurately measure ejection fraction and detect regional and global myocardial dysfunction.

3. therapy

Treatment is the same as for congestive cardiomyopathy of any cause. There is no specific therapy for myocardial damage caused by radiation or chemotherapy.

Cardiac dysrhythmias

1. etiology

(a) Anthracycline antibiotics cause dysrhythmias unrelated to the cumulative dose; these effects may appear hours or days after administration.

Frequently observed rhythm disturbances include supraventricular tachycardia, complete heart block and ventricular tachycardia. Doxorubicin may also prolong the QT interval.

(b) Amacrine causes ventricular dysrhythmias.

(c) Taxol causes bradycardia and may cause ventricular tachycardia when combined with cisplatin.

2. Diagnosis and treatment are the same as in rhythm disturbances of other etiology.

Superior vena cava syndrome (EVS)

Aetiology: Disruption of blood flow from the superior vena cava to the right atrium caused by extravascular compression or intravascular obstruction.

a) In 95 percent of cases, the cause is external compression of the ERV by a malignant mediastinal tumor (3 percent - benign diseases).

(b) The most common tumors are bronchogenic small cell carcinoma (48%) and lymphoma (21%).

2. Clinical manifestations

(a) Shortness of breath that increases when lying on your back or leaning forward.

(b) Tachypnea and signs of airway obstruction.

c) Signs and symptoms of increased intracranial pressure (e.g., dizziness, headache, visual disturbance, seizures, mental status changes).

d) Dysphagia, hoarseness.

(e) Dilation of veins in the neck, pallor of the face, and edema.

f) Numerous, dilated, vertically oriented and tortuous skin venules or veins above the edge of the thorax.

g) Swelling of the upper body, cyanosis and ruddy complexion.

(h) The immediate causes of death are airway obstruction and intracranial hemorrhage. Thrombosis of the ERV can occur in 30% of such patients.

3. Diagnostics

a) Clinical suspicion.

b) Computed tomography with intravenous contrast is the diagnostic procedure of choice.

(c) Transesophageal echocardiography is a safe procedure at the patient's bedside that is excellent for evaluation of the ER and surrounding structures.

(d) Angiography and radionuclide venography help localize the obstruction.

4. therapy

a) Symptomatic relief is the rule.

(b) Surgical bypass surgery relieves symptoms faster than radiation and is indicated in patients with life-threatening respiratory distress or progressive cerebral edema.

(c) Endovascular therapy (stents) has been successfully tested on many patients.

(d) Radiation therapy is the primary treatment for most malignant ERV obstructions; although in small cell carcinoma and lymphoma, chemotherapy is particularly useful.

(e) Temporary measures may be used in patients without significant airway obstruction or neurologic impairment and include corticosteroids to reduce cerebral and laryngeal edema, diuretics, and head elevation.

f) Anticoagulation does not play a definitive role.

Gastroenterology

Neutropenic enterocolitis (ileocecal syndrome or typhlitis)

1. Morbidity

Neutropenic enterocolitis usually occurs in patients with malignant hematologic diseases (leukemia is the most common disease, with an incidence of 10-40%) receiving chemotherapy.

2. Pathophysiology

Neutropenic enterocolitis results from mucosal ulceration and mucosal necrosis of the ileum, rectum or ascending colon with excessive growth and wall invasion by bacteria and/or fungi. Thrombocytopenia may predispose patients to hemorrhage in the intestinal wall. Enterocolitis usually presents on the seventh day of severe neutropenia.

3. Clinical manifestations

(a) Bloating of the abdomen

(b) Soreness in the right side of the abdomen

(c) watery diarrhea

(d) fever

(e) Thrombocytopenia and neutropenia

4. Diagnostics

a) Clinical suspicion.

(b) Routine abdominal radiographs may show ileus
with rectal distension and intestinal pneumatosis.

c) Abdominal computed tomography: Thickened intestinal wall containing air.

(d) Sigmoidoscopy.

5. Differential diagnosis

(a) appendicitis

(b) Pseudomembranous colitis

(c) Diverticulitis

(d) Other acute abdominal illnesses

6. Medical therapy

(a) Nutritional support

(b) Nasogastric aspiration

(c) Broad-spectrum antibiotics covering anaerobic, gram-negative bacteria and Clostridium difficile

7. Indications for surgical intervention

a) Perforation

b) Heavy bleeding

(c) Abscess

(d) Uncontrolled sepsis

e) No improvement after 2-3 days of intensive conservative treatment.

Bleeding and perforation of the gastrointestinal tract (GIT)

1. Bleeding from the GI tract

a) The most common cause is hemorrhagic gastritis (32-48%), followed by peptic ulcer disease.

(b) Only 12-17% of bleeding is caused by a tumor per se (most commonly seen in gastrointestinal lymphomas).

(c) Less common causes include esophageal varices, Mallory-Weiss tears, candidiasis esophagitis, and enteritis.

2. Perforation

Lymphomas are the most common malignancies that result in perforation during chemotherapy.

3. Diagnostics

A standard diagnostic examination should be performed to identify the source of bleeding, with an emphasis on endoscopy.

4. therapy

(a) Surgical

(b) Temporary methods of controlling bleeding include:

1. angiography, with or without embolization.

2. endoscopic intervention.

3 These methods may also be useful for patients with carcinomatosis and previously unresectable disease.

Renal function/metabolic disorders

Many cancer patients develop metabolic abnormalities caused by factors produced by the tumor (hormones or topical substances) or by tumor destruction as a result of antineoplastic therapy.

Hypercalcemia

1. Causes of hypercalcemia in cancer patients

a) Secondary to a malignant tumor 4%

(b) Etiology other than malignancy 77%

c) With concomitant hyperparathyroidism 2%.

d) Vitamin D intoxication 16%

e) Idiopathic

2. it is the most common metabolic abnormality in cancer patients (10%).

3. can occur with or without bone metastases.

4. Breast cancer is associated with hypercalcemia in 27-35% of patients.   Mechanisms include widespread osteolytic metastases, parathyroid hormone production, prostaglandin E2 (PGE2) (after hormone therapy with estrogens or anti-estrogens), humoral osteoclast-activating factor, and concomitant primary hyperparathyroidism.

5. Lung cancer is associated with hypercalcemia in 12.5-35% of patients. It is common in squamous cell carcinoma, carcinoma, and rarely in small cell carcinoma. It can occur early or late, with or without bone

metastases. Mechanisms include production of osteoclast-activating factor, transforming growth factor alpha, interleukin 1, and tumor necrosis factor.

6. Multiple myeloma causes hypercalcemia in 20-40% of patients. Hypercalcemia develops secondary to extensive osteolytic bone destruction, osteoclast-activating factor, and lymphotoxin. Fifty percent develop renal failure, which may exacerbate the hypercalcemia.

7. Lymphoma causes hypercalcemia through humoral mediation and local bone destruction.

8. Malignant head and neck tumors have a 6% incidence of hypercalcemia, which is humorally mediated.
Hypercalcemia was associated with malignant tumors of the oropharynx (37%), hypopharynx (24.3%), and tongue (21.5%).

9. Squamous cell, transitional cell, bladder, kidney, and ovarian carcinomas can also cause humoral hypercalcemia.

10. Clinical picture

(a) The severity of the disease depends on the degree of hypercalcemia, comorbidities or weaknesses, age, and concomitant metabolic disorders.

(b) Hypercalcemia in malignant tumors usually has a rapid onset.

(c) Neuromuscular manifestations often predominate and include lethargy, confusion, stupor and coma (occurs with serum calcium levels >13 mg/dL). Hallucinations and psychosis, weakness and decreased deep tendon reflexes (DTRs) are also common.

(d) Cardiovascular manifestations include increased cardiac contractility, hypersensitivity to digitalis, and arrhythmias.

e) Renal manifestations include polyuria and polydipsia (the earliest symptoms), dehydration, decreased glomerular filtration, loss of concentrating capacity, and renal failure.

(f) Gastrointestinal signs and symptoms include nausea and vomiting, anorexia, obstipation/ constipation, ileus, and abdominal pain.

(g) Skeletal damage is the hallmark of hypercalcemia caused by osteolytic metastases or humoral-mediated bone resorption leading to pain, abnormal fractures, deformity or necrosis.

11. Diagnosis

(a) Laboratory tests.

Total and ionized serum calcium

Electrolytes, serum urea nitrogen, and creatinine

3. Serum phosphorus and alkaline phosphatase

Measurement of urinary calcium and cyclic adenosine monophosphate (cAMP) excretion

5. High level of alkaline phosphatase

6. Increased calcium excretion in the urine

(b) Radiological studies.

1. Radionuclide bone scan

2. skeletal examination

3. basic chest radiography

c) ECG should be performed, paying attention to characteristic changes, including prolongation of PR and QRS intervals, shortened QT.

12. treatment

Hypercalcemia is often fatal if left untreated, especially when symptoms are present or when serum calcium is >13 mg/dL. Treatment goals include stimulating urinary calcium excretion, inhibiting bone resorption, and reducing calcium intake into the extracellular fluid.

a) Hydration: to restore intravascular volume and increase urine flow.

1. Initially 5-8 L of normal saline intravenously for the first 24 hours, followed by intravenous administration of sufficient fluids to maintain urine output at 3-4 L/day.

2. Electrolytes should be monitored during the infusion of saline.

3. Monitor urine and cardiac status to avoid fluid overload.

(b) Diuretics: Loop diuretics, such as furosemide, promote calciuresis by blocking calcium reabsorption in the ascending loop of the Genle, and enhance the calciuretic effect of normal saline.

1. Furosemide at a dose of 40-80 mg intravenously may be after adequate hydration.

2. Monitor electrolytes and urine output to avoid hyperdiuresis.

(c) Bone resorption inhibitors should be started for symptomatic hypercalcemia.

1. Mitramycin is an antitumor antibiotic with a direct toxic effect on osteoclasts. The usual dose is 25 µg/kg intravenously for 6 h. It usually reduces serum calcium within 6-48 h; it can be repeated if the patient does not respond within 2 days. Use should be limited to emergency treatment of severe hypercalcemia.

Complications include thrombocytopenia, myelosuppression, hypotension, hepatic and renal toxicity.

2. sodium ethidronate (EHDP) is a pyrophosphate analog that blocks osteoclastic bone resorption and bone crystal formation. The dose is 7.5 mg/kg/day in 250 ml of saline, administered for 2-6 hours for 3-7 days, then 20 mg/kg/day orally. Onset of action is slow, normocalcemia is achieved after 4-7 days in 75% of cases. EHDP is contraindicated in patients with renal insufficiency.

3. Glucocorticoids (e.g., prednisone) are most effective in hematological malignancies (especially multiple myeloma) and breast

carcinoma, and are ineffective in solid tumors. These drugs reduce serum calcium levels by inhibiting calcium absorption and vitamin D action.

Prednisone at a dose of 1-2 mg/kg/day starts to work after 3-5 days. Adverse effects include GI bleeding, hyperglycemia, and osteopenia.

4. Calcitonin inhibits osteoclastic bone resorption and enhances calcium excretion. The dose is 4-8 IU/kg every 6 hours intravenously or intraosseously. It can reduce calcium levels by 2-3 mg/dL over 2-3 hours. Adverse reactions include nausea and vomiting, hyperemia, and hypersensitivity reactions (prior skin testing is recommended before administration).

(d) Hemodialysis is useful for patients who have renal failure or who cannot be treated with forced diuresis.

(e) Specific antineoplastic therapy should be initiated in patients for whom a cure exists. It is the most effective means of achieving long-term correction of cancer-related hypercalcemia.

Tumor lysis syndrome. Tumor lysis syndrome is observed when cytotoxic chemotherapy causes rapid lysis of tumor cells in patients with a large number of malignant cells sensitive to tumor chemotherapy. Intracellular metabolites are released in amounts that exceed the excretory capacity of the kidneys.

1 This syndrome classically occurs in patients with Burkitt's lymphoma and non-Hodgkin's lymphoma, acute lymphoblastic and non-lymphoblastic leukemia, and chronic myelogenous leukemia.

2. May occur spontaneously in patients with lymphoma and leukemia or after treatment with chemotherapy, radiation, glucocorticoids, tamoxifen and/or interferon.

3. Manifestations

a) Related to metabolic disorders

1. Hyperkalemia: generalized weakness, irritability, decreased deep tendon reflexes (DTRs), paresthesias, paralysis, cardiac dysrhythmias, and cardiac arrest. Classic ECG changes include peak T waves, reduced R waves progressing to dilated QRS, prolonged PR, loss of P wave, and a sinusoidal pattern as the final event.

2. Hypocalcemia (associated with hyperphosphatemia): muscle cramps, carpopedal cramps, facial grimaces, laryngeal spasm, irritability, depression, psychosis, intestinal cramps, chronic malabsorption, seizures and respiratory arrest. Signs of Chvostek and signs of Trousseau are present in some patients. An ECG reveals a prolonged QT interval.

3. Hyperuricemia: gouty arthritis, nephrolithiasis and urate nephropathy.

(b) Precipitation of calcium salts in tissues

c) Acute renal failure

4. Prevention and treatment

a) To prevent acute renal failure, patients undergoing treatment for malignant neoplasms should receive

I. In the absence of metabolic aberrations:

1. Allopurinol 500 mg/m^2 BSA/day; reduce to 200 mg/m^2 BSA/day, 3 days after starting chemotherapy

2. Hydration, 3000 ml/m^2 BSA/day

3 Chemotherapy should be started within 24-48 hours of admission.

4. Monitoring of electrolytes, urea, creatinine, uric acid, calcium, phosphorus every 12-14 h.

II. When there are metabolic abnormalities:

Allopurinol start as above, reduce dose if hyperuricemia is controlled, reduce dose if renal insufficiency.

2. Hydration as above, add non-thiazide diuretics if necessary.

3. Urine alkalization (urine pH >7)

Sodium bicarbonate 100 mEq/L intravenously at first, adjust as needed. Cancel when uric acid becomes normal.

4. chemotherapy is delayed until uric acid is normal or until dialysis is started.

5. Do the same tests every 6-12 hours until stabilized (at least for 3-5 days)

6. Replace calcium with Ca^{++} gluconate by slow intravenous infusion in case of symptomatic hypocalcemia or severe ECG changes

7. Treat hyperkalemia with exchange resins, bicarbonate.

III. Criteria for hemodialysis in patients not responding to the above measures:

1. Serum potassium $\geq$6 mEq/L

2. Serum uric acid $\geq$10 mg/dL

3. rapidly increasing serum phosphorus or $\geq$10 mg/dL

4. Liquid overloading

5. Symptomatic hypocalcemia

Body surface area BSA 1. Vigorous intravenous hydration, often with diuretics or a renal dose of dopamine to ensure adequate urine excretion

2. urine alkalization during the first 1-2 days of cytotoxic therapy to increase uric acid solubility

Allopurinol to reduce uric acid formation

Other common metabolic disorders in cancer

1. Syndrome of Inadequate Secretion of Antidiuretic Hormone (SIADH)

a) Occurs in 1-2% of cancer patients

(b) Prevalent in small cell carcinoma of the lung, as well as in prostate, pancreatic, ureteric, and bladder cancer

(c) Sometimes found in lymphomas and leukemias.

2. Hypoglycemia

a) Insulinomas: benign islet cell tumors that secrete insulin

b) Non-islet cell tumors (e.g., mesothelioma, fibrosarcoma, hemangiopericytoma, hepatoma, adrenocortical carcinoma, leukemia and lymphoma, pseudomyxoma, pheochromocytoma, anaplastic carcinoma)

Hematology

Cancer itself, antineoplastic therapy, and acute conditions occurring in cancer patients result in hematologic abnormalities. Red blood cells, white blood cells, platelets and clotting factors can be affected quantitatively, qualitatively or both. Bleeding and infection are major life-threatening events in critically ill cancer patients, and they are both the cause and result of hematologic abnormalities.

Evidence-Based Practice of Critical Care, 3rd Edition *Authors: Clifford S. Deutschman & Patrick J. Neligan*

CHAPTER 2. CHEMOTHERAPY-INDUCED HYPERSENSITIVITY. MANAGEMENT OF INFUSION REACTIONS TO SYSTEMIC ANTICANCER THERAPY: ESMO CLINICAL GUIDELINES

Most anticancer drugs are associated with a risk of infusion reactions (IRs); the incidence may increase with concomitant use of different agents. IRs are either allergic reactions to foreign proteins (usually immunoglobulin E (IgE)-mediated allergic reactions) or non-immune-mediated reactions. Most IRs are mild with symptoms such as chills, fever, nausea, headache, skin rash, itching, etc. Severe reactions are less common and can be fatal without appropriate intervention. IRs are "type B" reactions: they are dose-independent, unpredictable, usually unrelated to the pharmacological activity of the drug, and usually go away after stopping treatment. These reactions are divided into true allergic reactions (immune-mediated, such as anaphylactic reactions) and nonallergic (nonimmune) sensitivity reactions. Gell and Coombs defined the classification of type B adverse reactions to therapeutic agents as the four states of true hypersensitivity. Adverse nonimmune type B reactions include: pseudoallergic [anaphylactoid reactions that resemble true type I reactions with direct mast cell degranulation, such as cytokine release syndrome (CRS)], idiosyncrasic reactions (unusual, unpredictable, unrelated to the pharmacological action of the drug). and intolerances.

Reactions

Etiology and manifestation

Asparaginase has the highest rate of hypersensitivity reactions (6-43%). The incidence is higher when the drug is administered intravenously and as a single agent. Usually after several doses within 1 h of drug administration. Common manifestations include:

(a) Hypotension or hypertension.

(b) Laryngospasm and respiratory distress. Agitation.

(c) Facial edema. Reactions can be life-threatening and are more likely to occur after 2 or more weeks of treatment.

Prophylaxis: corticosteroids and antihistamines.

2. Cisplatin is the second most common antineoplastic drug causing hypersensitivity reactions (1-20%). Potentially fatal reactions occur in 5% of patients. An interval of repeated treatment >2 years increases the risk of developing a hypersensitivity reaction (HRR). Patients receiving an eighth course of carboplatin or a second dose after reintroduction of the drug should be particularly cautious. Oxaliplatin causes acute RGH in 0.5-25% of cases, and the maximum reaction occurs on the seventh to eighth dose. Skin tests can predict reactions to carboplatin. A negative skin test appears to be reasonably reliable in predicting the absence of severe RGH on subsequent administration of the drug. The first RGH on oxaliplatin is usually mild, but may become more severe with repeated administration. Approximately 50% of patients re-treated with platinum drugs experience a recurrence of RGH despite premedication.

Desensitization protocols are optional. Corticosteroids and H1/H2 antagonists are not usually recommended. *Premedication cannot prevent IR.* For patients who develop acute laryngopharyngeal dysesthesia during or after oxaliplatin infusion, treatment by heating the air the patient is breathing is sufficient to improve symptoms, and no other measures are required.

Alkylating agents are much less likely to cause hypersensitivity reactions.

a) Melphalan causes anaphylactic reactions in about 2-3% of patients.

b) Bleomycin causes a febrile state in 20-25% of patients, which in some cases develops into a life-threatening syndrome (confusion, chills, respiratory distress, hypotension), especially when administered intravenously to patients with lymphoma. Develops immediately or with a delay of several hours, usually after the first or second dose. If anaphylactoid reaction occurs, patients with lymphoma should be given 2 units or less for the first 2 doses. If IR does not occur, the normal dosing schedule can be followed.

c) Doxorubicin can also cause anaphylaxis. Premedication is not recommended.

d) Docetaxel. 30% of reactions without premedication, 2% of severe reactions with premedication. First or second dose, within the first 10 min of infusion. Prophylaxis: oral dexamethasone 8 mg twice daily for 3 days (starting 1 day before taking docetaxel).

e) Etoposide. Anaphylactic reactions 1%-3%. Usually after 1 dose. Slow infusion for 30-60 min. Corticosteroids and antihistamines for prophylaxis.

f) Paclitaxel. 30% IRs without premedication. Severe anaphylactic reaction in 2%-4%. First or second dose, within the first 10 min of infusion. Prophylaxis: one dose of intravenous dexamethasone plus diphenhydramine (50 mg intravenously) and an H_2 -receptor antagonist (ranitidine 50 mg or cimetidine 300 mg intravenously) 30 min before infusion of paclitaxel.

g) MoAb monoclonal antibodies are non-endogenous proteins that can provoke all four types of reactions. The incidence of IR with the first administration of MoAb ranges from 77% for rituximab, 40% for trastuzumab, to 15% for cetuximab. The likelihood of IR decreases with each subsequent course of therapy. A distinctive side effect of MoAb is the possibility of non-allergic IR caused by cytokine release during the first hours after infusion. It is believed that the interaction of MoAbs with the target can lead to the release of cytokines that cause a number of symptoms similar to those seen in type I allergic reactions. Unlike Type I reactions, the symptoms disappear with each successive dose.

h)   Ofatumumumab. 61%, the majority more often on the first injection. Premedication 30 min to 2 h before defatumumumab: oral paracetamol 1 g, oral or intravenous antihistamine (e.g., diphenhydramine 50 mg or cetirizine 10 mg), intravenous corticosteroid (prednisolone: for previously untreated or recurrent CLL 50 mg and for refractory CLL 100 mg). If the patient is not experiencing IR, the first and second corticosteroid infusions may be reduced or absent altogether.

Therapy

Stop the infusion

✓ Maintain intravenous access

✓ DDC assessment: airway, breathing, circulation

✓ Assess the level of consciousness and vital signs

✓ Position: in case of arterial hypotension, the patient should be transferred to Trendelenburg position; in case of respiratory failure, the patient should sit up; and, if unconscious, the patient should be placed in the recovery position.

Severe reactions (suspected anaphylaxis and acute onset of respiratory symptoms and/or hypotension)

a) Stop the infusion of the antineoplastic drug immediately.

(b) Epinephrine 0.5-0.75 ml (1:1000 in 10 ml of normal saline) administered intravenously every 5-15 minutes.

In hypotension:

- dopamine 400 mg in 500 ml at a rate of 2-20 mcg/kg/min or

- vasopressin 25 IU in 250 ml of 5% DV or NS (0.1 IU/ml), dose 0.01-0.04 IU/min

(c) Normal saline 1-2 L intravenous infusion at a rate of 5-10 ml/kg for the first 5 minutes. Aminophylline in acute bronchospasm. In bradycardia atropine 600 mcg v/v.

(d) Diphenhydramine (or other antihistamines) 25-50 mg intravenously plus ranitidine 50 mg intravenously.

Corticosteroids are effective in preventing biphasic reactions, but are not critical in the treatment of anaphylaxis. Hydrocortisone 500 mg intravenously initially and repeatedly every 6 hours for prolonged reactions. The corticosteroid dose is equivalent to 1-2 mg/kg w/v (methyl)prednisolone every 6 hours.

2. For non-serious reactions (when cytokine release is suspected)-low rate/short termination of *infusion*

Treatment:

✓ H1/H2 antagonists: diphenhydramine 50 mg intravenously plus ranitidine 50 mg intravenously

✓ Hydrocortisone 500 mg intravenously initially and repeatedly every 6 hours for prolonged reactions. The corticosteroid dose is equivalent to 1-2 mg/kg w/v (methyl)prednisolone every 6 hours.

✓ Restart infusion at 50% and titrate to tolerable 3/4: stop infusion if reaction-repeat treatment.

✓ Post-reaction: basic vital signs should be monitored and symptoms of relapse should be controlled.

✓ After a severe reaction, close observation for 24 hours is recommended.

Immunocompromised

A patient with cancer (especially during chemotherapy) should be considered an immunocompromised patient.

Types of immune defects recognized in cancer patients

1. Defects of cellular and humoral immunity

a) Defective mononuclear phagocyte T-lymphocytes: Hodgkin's disease, lymphoma and cytotoxic chemotherapy

(b) Decreased or absent B-cell function in patients with multiple myeloma and chronic lymphocytic leukemia

2. Neutropenia

(a) Neutropenia is the most common immunological defect in patients with neoplastic diseases.

(b) The risk of bacteremia and fungal infection is increased when the absolute neutrophil count (ANC) is <1000/mm^3 .

c) Myelotoxic chemotherapy is the most common cause of neutropenia; neutropenia is also seen in leukemia, aplastic anemia, drug reactions, and when bone marrow is destroyed by a tumor or radiation.

Treatment of febrile neutropenia: ESMO clinical guidelines

Febrile neutropenia (FN) is defined as an oral temperature >38.3°C or two consecutive measurements >38.0°C within 2 h and an absolute neutrophil count (ANC) <0.5 × 10^9 /L, or expected to fall below 0.5 × 10^9 /L. Most standard-dose CT regimens are associated with neutropenia within 6 to 8 days, and FN is observed in~8 cases per 1,000 patients receiving oncologic CT. Several factors other than CT itself have been shown to be responsible for the increased risk of FN and its complications. Among them, age, advanced disease, previous FN, lack of antibiotic prophylaxis or use of granulocyte colony-stimulating factor, mucositis, poor performance and/or cardiovascular disease play a major role. EORTC (European Organization for Research and Treatment of Cancer) and American Society of Clinical Oncology (ASCO) guidelines recommend that clinicians limit the use of antibiotic prophylaxis to patients at high risk of FN; others recommend simply avoiding such practices to prevent FN. The most recent Cochrane meta-analysis update still recommended the use of ciprofloxacin or levofloxacin in cancer patients undergoing intensive CT. A recent meta-analysis of randomized controlled trials and real-world experience confirm the outstanding (> 50% success rate) of primary prophylaxis with filgrastim or pegfilgrastim.

Main recommendations for maintaining the FN

✓ FN is seen in ±1% of patients receiving CT; this is associated with significant morbidity (20-30%) and mortality (10%).

✓ FN can be effectively prevented with G-CSF; it is recommended that these drugs be used in patients receiving chemotherapy with a risk of FN >20%, and in patients with serious comorbidities and/or >60 years of age [I, A]

✓ Patients with FN should be evaluated for risk of complications using the MASCC scale [I, A].

✓ Patients with FN at low risk of complications can often be treated with oral antibiotics and possibly on an outpatient basis if adequate follow-up is available [I, A]

✓ Patients with FN at high risk of complications should be hospitalized and treated promptly with broad-spectrum antibiotics; these patients should be closely monitored for instability (before shock) [I, A]

In addition to standard treatment with broad-spectrum antibacterials, there are a number of situations in clinical practice that require a specific regimen. The duration of treatment may vary, and in these circumstances, local recommendations for antibiotic therapy should be followed. If the patient has an intravenous catheter, a catheter-related infection (CRI) should be suspected, and blood cultures from the catheter and peripheral vessels should be performed. Glycopeptides such as vancomycin should be administered through the catheter whenever possible to cover Gram-positive microorganisms. Teicoplanin is a useful alternative because it can be administered once daily. Consultation with a clinical microbiologist is recommended, along with appropriate therapy against infection with fungi or pneumocysts. The choice of antifungal drugs will depend on individual patient characteristics and the use of prior prophylactic therapy. Therapy for suspected aspergillosis (for cases with typical CT infiltrates) may consist of either voriconazole or liposomal amphotericin B. These antifungals can be combined with echinocandin for resistant disease. In patients with suspected invasive fungal infection, an accurate microbiological diagnosis is highly desirable. High-dose co-trimoxazole is the drug of choice in suspected pneumocystinfections. The addition of vancomycin extends protection against cutaneous pathogens. Linezolid and daptomycin are new alternatives to glycopeptides; however, additional clinical experience is needed, especially in patients with neutropenia. If there are clinical or microbiologic signs of intra-abdominal or pelvic sepsis, treatment with metronidazole should be initiated unless the patient is on carbapenem or piperacillin-tazobactam, which have adequate anaerobic action. Empirical initiation of antifungal therapy is recommended for patients whose fever is not treatable with broad-spectrum antibiotics after 3 to 7 days of appropriate treatment. A CT scan of the liver and spleen should be performed before initiation of antifungal therapy. Fluconazole can be administered as a first-line treatment if the patient has a low risk of invasive aspergillosis. Initial antifungal treatment should be continued until neutropenia disappears or for at least 14 days in patients with confirmed invasive candidiasis infection. Daily evaluation of fever trends, bone marrow function, and renal function is indicated until the patient's fever disappears and ANC, absolute neutrophil count $\geq 0.5 \times 10^9$ /l within 24 hours is achieved. Repeated imaging may be required in patients with persistent fever.

If the patient has no fever and ANC $\geq 0.5 \times 10^9$ /L after 48 h, has low risk, and the cause of infection is not detected, consider switching to oral antibiotics. If the patient is at high risk and the cause is not found and is on dual therapy, aminoglycosides may be discontinued. When the cause is found, continue appropriate specific therapy.

If the patient's fever persists after 48 hours but is clinically stable, initial antibiotic therapy should be continued. If the patient is clinically unstable, antibiotic therapy should be alternated or expanded if justified by clinical development.

Violation of the integrity of tissues or mucous membranes

a) Diagnostic procedures including skin puncture and biopsies

b) Invasive procedures, such as placing central venous catheters and pulmonary artery catheters, urinary catheters, or endotracheal tubes

c) Loss of physical, chemical, and immunological barrier functions of the intestinal mucosa

4. Hyposplenic or post-splenectomy conditions

a) Reduced body response to infections caused by encapsulated organisms such as S. pneumoniae, Haemophilus influenza and Neisseria meningitides.

Clinical evaluation

A careful review of the medical history of the patient who received antineoplastic drugs.

2. examine recurrent infections, exposure to contagious diseases, and recent travel.

3. The presence of fever without an obvious source should be carefully examined by evaluating the following:

(a) Blood, urine, and sputum

(b) Intubation catheters

(c) Surgical or other skin wounds

(d) Cerebrospinal fluid (CSF)

(e) feces

f) Possibility of non-drained accumulations and abscesses

4. Skin lesions should be carefully examined. Ecthyma gangrenosum is a characteristic skin lesion associated with bacterial and fungal sepsis.

5. The oral cavity is another potential source of infection in immunocompromised individuals. Sinusitis and periodontitis can be sources, especially in orotracheally or nasotracheally intubated patients and patients with nasogastric tubes.

6. Funduscopic examination is necessary to detect fungal infection, especially in patients with central venous and urinary catheters.

7. Perianal lesions can cause severe infection.

8. Panoculture is indicated in all febrile patients. All vascular catheters should be removed and replaced.

Literature:

- ✓ Management of infusion reactions to systemic anticancer therapy: ESMO Clinical Practice Guidelines. Annals of Oncology 28 (Supplement 4): iv100-iv118, 2017 doi:10.1093/annonc/mdx216.
- ✓ Management of febrile neutropaenia: ESMO Clinical Practice Guidelines Annals of Oncology 27 (Supdpolie:1m0e.1nt059)3:/va1n1n1o-nvc1/1m8d,w2302156

CHAPTER 3. ONCOLOGY EMERGENCIES

Cancer emergencies are subdivided into:

(a) Structural or compressive due to a tumor mass,

b) metabolic or hormonal

c) caused by the ongoing treatment.

Structural and obstructive cancer emergencies

Cardiac tamponade

Patients may present with chest pain, shortness of breath or difficulty breathing, orthopnea, hypotension, or even shock. Examination reveals tachycardia, dilated jugular veins, facial edema, hypotension, paradoxical pulse and muffled heart murmurs. Only a few patients present with the classic Beck triad. Cardiac tamponade results from either a blockage in the lymphatic drainage or from lesions in the pericardium. This can occur as a result of nonmalignant conditions such as uremia, infections, concomitant autoimmune diseases, or as a result of radiation pericarditis, acute or chronic. Malignant conditions that can cause cardiac tamponade are lung cancer, mediastinal lymphoma, breast cancer, or melanoma. Primary cardiac malignancies, such as mesothelioma, are very rare. Echocardiography (ECHO) is usually the tool to diagnose cardiac tamponade. Pericardiocentesis and urgent fluid removal will relieve the symptoms. The fluid should always be sent for malignant cytology. Treatment includes elimination of the underlying cause, pericardiocentesis, or pericardial removal if radiation-induced chronic pericarditis is the cause. Sclerosing agents such as bleomycin and tetracyclines may be used in conjunction with pericardiocentesis.

Superior vena cava syndrome (CVS)

Patients experience headache, puffiness of the face, swelling around the eyes, difficulty breathing when lying down or leaning forward, nasal bleeding (epistaxis), or even hoarseness of the voice.

These symptoms increase when lying down, leaning forward, coughing, or sneezing. Examination reveals edema, sometimes even of the hands, swollen jugular veins, venous dilation in the chest and upper arms, proptosis or stridor.

This occurs as a result of compression, invasion, thrombosis or fibrosis of the large veins in the head, neck and upper extremities of the body. Usually the obstruction develops unnoticed and collaterals are formed, so it is rare for an emergency condition to occur. Cancers that lead to superior vena cava syndrome are usually lymphomas, lung cancer, especially squamous cell and small cell, breast cancer, especially right-sided, germ cell tumors and thymomas.

The most common cancer is lung cancer, whereas embryonal cell tumors and thymomas account for less than 2% of the causes of superior vena cava obstruction. Upper vena cava obstruction can also result from central lines established in the internal jugular veins. Nononcologic causes of superior vena cava obstruction syndrome include sarcoidosis, tuberculosis, retrosternal goiter, and idiopathic mediastinal fibrosis. It can also occur as a long-term consequence of radiation therapy.

Superior vena cava syndrome is a clinical diagnosis. A chest computed tomography (CT) scan can help identify the location of the obstruction and the presence of collaterals, if any.

Because superior vena cava syndrome usually presents before a cancer diagnosis, a CT scan will also help in determining where to biopsy the tumor. In pediatric patients, it is important to remember that anesthesia for biopsy may result in difficult or prolonged intubation due to tumor compression of the small airways.

Bone marrow study for staging of the disease may have to be delayed until the patient is stabilized. The treatment of superior vena cava syndrome is to start cancer therapy. Radiation therapy is not used routinely anymore. Most patients respond to steroids, which are used to treat cancer as well as to reduce swelling. If a thrombus is present, the central catheters should be removed and anticoagulation or thrombolytic therapy should be started.

Thrombolytic therapy should not be used unless metastasis to the brain has been ruled out. Radiation therapy is used for those patients who have failed chemotherapy, especially in cases of small cell lung cancer.

Stenting of the superior vena cava can be used in those who have failed chemotherapy or radiation therapy. The stent will relieve the symptoms immediately, but remains for the rest of the patient's life.

Step 1: Algorithm for resuming airway obstruction requiring intubation (using a small endotracheal tube) and ventilation before definitive treatment. Position on a stand to facilitate venous drainage. Do not give intravenous or intramuscular injections into the upper extremity.

Step 2: Do the visualization

- Computed tomography (CT) of the chest with or without venography

- These patients may not be able to lie in a horizontal position for a chest CT

- They should be intubated before CT or empirical therapy should be started

- Upper extremity venogram or duplex ultrasound for patients with a central venous catheter in the upper extremity to rule out venous thrombus.

Step 3: Confirming the diagnosis

- Perform a biopsy before starting therapy if the diagnosis is unclear. Correct

Appropriate hemostatic measures should be taken when performing invasive procedures.

- Current treatment guidelines emphasize the importance of an accurate histologic diagnosis before initiating therapy

Step 4: Chemotherapy and corticosteroids

- They can be used, especially in chemo/steroid-sensitive tumors.

Step 5: Radiotherapy

- This is the standard treatment for sensitive tumors, but it may take several weeks for the effects to appear. Steroids are usually used to prevent post-radiation edema, especially if there is pre-existing laryngeal edema.

- In most cases, emergency RT is no longer considered necessary on admission.

Step 6: Stenting the superior vena cava

- The efficacy and ability to alleviate symptoms of superior vena cava syndrome has been proven.

- Current guidelines recommend an endovascular approach initially in patients with severe symptoms. (Strydor due to central airway obstruction, laryngeal edema, coma due to cerebral edema).

Step 7: Thrombolysis and prolonged anticoagulation

- Endovascular techniques serve as a "rescue" strategy for patients with life-threatening symptoms such as cerebral edema, laryngeal edema or hemodynamic shock. They usually avoid surgical intervention in patients with limited life expectancy.

- Patients with extensive thrombosis or stenotic lesions may be considered for local catheter-directed thrombolysis or mechanical endovascular thrombectomy.

Step 8: Surgical treatment

- Surgical treatment should be considered in patients with malignant thymoma, thymic carcinoma, and in selected patients with non-small cell lung cancer along with other adjuvant therapies.

Urinary tract obstruction

Urinary tract obstruction is manifested by pain in the abdomen or side,

decreased urination or anuria. The patient may be anasarca due to fluid retention. Urinary tract obstruction is caused by urologic or gynecologic cancers or even in cases of abdominal lymphoma.

Computed tomography to diagnose the site of the obstruction and to take a biopsy may be helpful. Percutaneous nephrostomy or suprapubic drainage may be placed to relieve the obstruction. Anuria is often accompanied by polyuria, so dehydration and electrolyte imbalances should be closely monitored.

Increased intracranial pressure

Patients may come in with headaches, visual disturbances, strabismus, or even seizures. On examination, the patient may have altered breathing, strabismus, or papilledema. The 6th cranial nerve is most often involved. Manifestations depend on the size of the lesion. Increased ICP is usually caused by primary tumors or brain metastases. Metastases occur in the brain basins and in the gray-white matter. Primary intracranial tumors such as medulloblastomas or gliomas, as well as metastases from tumors such as breast, melanoma and renal cell carcinoma are important causes of elevated ICP. Not only a tumor, but swelling can also lead to elevated BP. Consider causes such as thrombosis and cavernous sinus syndrome if the patient is already taking chemotherapy drugs, especially L-asparaginase. Although magnetic resonance imaging (MRI) of the brain is the study of choice, CT may be easier and faster if the patient is unstable. Venography is necessary if thrombosis is suspected.

Treatment usually consists of initiation of steroids, usually dexamethasone, mannitol or 3% saline. These measures should be started as soon as the clinical diagnosis of elevated IOP is made, even before radiological confirmation. Some patients will require fluid diversion in cases of hydrocephalus with placement of a ventriculoperitoneal shunt or ventriculoatrial shunt. Chemotherapy or radiotherapy may be given for metastases. Whole-brain irradiation is usually performed for

multiple metastases, while cyber-knife or radiosurgery can be used for single lesions.

Spinal cord compression

Spinal cord compression (SCC) is the most common condition.

Most cases are due to lung cancer or Hodgkin's lymphoma.

Step 1: Intensive care

Compression of the tracheobronchial tree causing airway

compression is an emergency airway aid requiring intubation (using a small endotracheal tube) and ventilation before definitive treatment. Position on a stand to facilitate venous drainage. Do not give intravenous or intramuscular injections into the upper extremity.

Step 2: Do the visualization

- Computed tomography (CT) of the chest with or without venography is the diagnosis of

- These patients may not be able to lie in a horizontal position for a chest CT

- They should be intubated before CT or empirical therapy should be started

- Upper extremity venogram or duplex ultrasound for patients with a central venous catheter in the upper extremity to rule out venous thrombus.

Step 3: Confirming the diagnosis

- Perform a biopsy before starting therapy if the diagnosis is unclear. Appropriate hemostatic measures should be taken when performing invasive procedures.

- Current treatment guidelines emphasize the importance of an accurate histologic diagnosis before initiating therapy.

Step 4: Chemotherapy and corticosteroids

- They can be used, especially in chemo/steroid-sensitive tumors.

Step 5: Radiotherapy

-This is the standard treatment for sensitive tumors, but it may take several weeks for the effects to appear. Steroids are usually used to prevent post-radiation edema, especially if there is pre-existing laryngeal edema.

- In most cases, emergency RT is no longer considered necessary on admission.

Step 6: Stenting the superior vena cava

- The efficacy and ability to alleviate symptoms of superior vena cava syndrome has been proven.

- Current guidelines recommend an endovascular approach initially in patients with severe symptoms. (Strydor due to central airway obstruction, laryngeal edema, coma due to cerebral edema).

Step 7: Thrombolysis and prolonged anticoagulation

- Endovascular techniques serve as a "rescue" strategy for patients with life-threatening symptoms such as cerebral edema, laryngeal edema. They usually avoid surgical intervention in patients with limited life expectancy.

- Patients with extensive thrombosis or stenotic lesions may considered for local catheter-directed thrombolysis or mechanical endovascular thrombectomy.

Step 8: Surgical treatment

- Surgical treatment should be considered in patients with malignant thymoma, thymic carcinoma, and selected patients with non-small cell lung cancer along with other adjuvant therapies

Urinary tract obstruction

Urinary tract obstruction is manifested by abdominal or flank pain, decreased urination or anuria. The patient may be anasarca due to fluid retention.

Urinary tract obstruction is caused by urologic or gynecologic cancers or even in cases of abdominal lymphoma.

Computed tomography to diagnose the site of the obstruction and to take a biopsy can be helpful.

Percutaneous nephrostomy or suprapubic drainage can be placed to relieve the obstruction. Anuria is often accompanied by polyuria, so dehydration and electrolyte imbalance should be closely monitored.

Increased intracranial pressure

Patients may come in with headaches, visual disturbances, strabismus, or even seizures. On examination, the patient may have altered breathing, strabismus, or papilledema. The 6th cranial nerve is most often involved. Manifestations depend on the size of the lesion. Elevated IOP is usually caused by primary brain tumors or brain metastases. Metastases occur in the watershed areas of the brain and in the gray-white matter.

Primary intracranial tumors such as medulloblastomas or gliomas as well as metastases of tumors such as breast, melanoma and renal cell carcinoma are important causes of elevated IOP. Not only a tumor, but swelling can also lead to elevated BP. Consider causes such as thrombosis and cavernous sinus syndrome if the patient is already taking chemotherapy drugs, especially L-asparaginase. Although magnetic resonance imaging (MRI) of the brain is the study of choice, CT may be easier and faster if the patient is unstable. Venography is necessary if thrombosis is suspected.

Treatment is usually initiation of steroids usually dexamethasone, mannitol, or 3% saline. These measures should be started as soon as the clinical diagnosis of elevated IOP is made, even before radiological confirmation. Some patients will require fluid diversion in cases of hydrocephalus with placement of a ventriculoperitoneal shunt or ventriculoatrial shunt. Chemotherapy or radiotherapy may be given for metastases. Whole-brain irradiation is usually done for multiple metastases, whereas cyber-knife or radiosurgery may be used for single lesions (up to 15).

Spinal cord compression

Spinal cord compression (SCC) is the most common cancer emergency requiring surgical intervention. It is defined as compression, displacement, or obstruction of the dural sac, which surrounds the spinal cord or cauda equina, in cancer. Patients have a history of back pain, tingling, numbness or weakness in the extremities, especially the lower extremities, or urinary and/or stool incontinence. Examination may reveal swelling in the back, spinal soreness, motor or sensory deficits in the extremities, hyperreflexia, positive Babinski's symptom, and decreased anal tone. The thoracic spine is the most common site of involvement, followed by the lumbosacral region. Cancers that can lead to SCC are metastases from breast, lung, prostate, non-Hodgkin's lymphoma; intraspinal spread of neuroblastoma or a skeletal lesion with melanoma causing vertebral collapse. An MRI of the spine helps delineate the focus of the lesion and plan therapy. If MRI is unavailable or contraindicated, computed tomographic myelography should be done. Treatment should be urgent, as delay may lead to permanent neurological damage. Treatment includes decompression with surgery, glucocorticoids, and radiation therapy (RT). Remote radiotherapy is usually preferred. There is no consensus on the dose of steroids, but higher doses may lead to more side effects such as gastritis, infections, or psychosis. Surgery is usually done if there is evidence of spinal instability. Spinal stability can be assessed using the Patchell scoring system. This assessment uses 6 criteria, namely tumor location, bone lesion quality (lytic/blastic/mixed), spinal alignment, vertebral body collapse, pain, and posterior spinal lesions.

Malignant compression of the spinal cord

A 68-year-old patient with prostate carcinoma presented with increasing back pain radiating to the right leg, accompanied by weakness and difficulty in walking and impaired bladder and bowel function.

Step 1: Intensive therapy

(a) Analgesia with adequate analgesics is a priority in these patients.

b) Immediate consultation with a neurosurgeon to save the limb

c) Special precautions must be taken when transporting these patients.

Step 2: Do imaging.

- In patients with a high index of suspicion and symptoms suggestive of bone metastasis, magnetic resonance imaging is the gold standard of diagnosis.

- An alternative is a CT scan of the spine.

- It is important to visualize the entire spine as several areas of compression may be present.

Step 3: Start with glucocorticoids

a) Dexamethasone is indicated in patients with movement disorders or radiological signs of nerve compression.

(b) It is administered as an initial intravenous dose of 10-16 mg and then 4 mg every 4 hours.

c) Ideally within 12 hours of onset of symptoms. Final therapy with radiation therapy or surgery should be introduced and steroids rapidly withdrawn, usually within 10-12 days.

d) Use proton pump inhibitors or H_2 -blockers along with high-dose corticosteroids.

Step 4: Consider surgery

It is indicated in most cases, especially in patients with good functional status. The indications are as follows: marked spinal instability, rapidly progressing symptoms, progressive symptoms during radiation therapy when tissue is needed for diagnosis, radiotherapy-resistant tumors.

Aggressive surgical treatment and postoperative LT should be considered for those with a more favorable prognosis or who are expected to have a possible neurologic recovery.

Step 5: consider radiation therapy

- This is the main treatment for patients with and without motor impairment.

- Usually combined with spinal stabilization surgery.

Step 6: consider chemohormonal therapy

- Hormonal chemotherapy and zoledronic acid should be considered for a sensitive tumor, such as prostate cancer, testicular tumor, or lymphoma.

Acute Airway Obstruction

Acute airway obstruction is said to occur when a patient has dyspnea and/or stridor. This may be the result of obstruction at or above the level of the main stem bronchi. If dyspnea occurs during exercise, it usually indicates that the airway diameter is less than 8 mm. If it occurs at rest, it suggests that the airway diameter is less than 5 mm. "Tracheal stenosis syndrome" refers to a cluster of symptoms consisting of shortness of breath, cough, wheezing, and stridor and is seen in approximately 85% of patients with primary tracheal tumors. Bleeding is seen in 45% of patients with obstructive neoplasms. Stridor is a threatening sign and requires urgent intervention.

Consider nonmalignant causes such as angioedema, infections, or foreign body aspiration, especially in children. Cancers that can cause acute airway obstruction are head and neck tumors and tumors arising from the lungs. Laryngoscopy and bronchoscopy can help identify lesions and for taking biopsies. Computed tomography to detect lower airway lesions. Steroids and radiation therapy are used to reduce obstruction. Stenting may be necessary if the lesion is external. Some centers may also use bronchoscopy with laser therapy or photodynamic therapy if the compression is internal.

Critical Care Medicine: An Algorithmic Approach, 1st Edition
Author : Alexander Goldfarb-Rumyantzev

METABOLIC OR HORMONAL EMERGENCIES

Carbohydrate emergencies include the following hyperglycemic conditions: diabetic ketoacidosis (DKA), hyperglycemic hyperosmolar state (HHS or HHS), and hypoglycemic emergencies.

Insulin deficiency, elevated levels of hormones that counteract insulin (cortisol, glucagon, growth hormone, and catecholamines), and peripheral insulin resistance leading to hyperglycemia, dehydration, ketosis, and electrolyte imbalance. DKA usually occurs in young patients with insulin-dependent type 1 diabetes, and GHS usually occurs in older people with type 2 diabetes either on oral hypoglycemic agents or insulin. The main pathophysiologic difference is the absence of circulating insulin in DKA and the presence of residual insulin function in HGS, which prevents lipolysis and ketosis.

Hyperglycemic Urgent Conditions

An 18-year-old female patient was admitted to the emergency department with high fever, tachypnea, and altered thinking. She had diarrhea for 3 days which was watery and large in volume. On examination, she was found to have a fever of 38.3 C° . Her pulse rate was 130 beats per minute and her blood pressure was 90/70 mmHg. She had a

Glasgow Coma Scale score of 9 and a glucose of 26.6 mmol/L on admission. There was no history of diabetes.

Differences between DKA and HHS

	Diabetic ketoacidosis	Hyperglycemic hyperosmolar syndrome
Ketoacidosis	Deep	Minimum or no
Glucose	~ 13.89 -33.3 mmol/l	Often >50 mmol/l
HCO3	<15 mEq/L	>15 mEq/L
Osmolarity	300-325 mOsm	Often >350 mOsm
Age	Young	The Elderly
Beginning	Acute; hours to days	Chronic; days to weeks
Related to Diabetes	Not always	Related
Cramps	Very seldom.	Often
Coma	Rarely	Often
Insulin levels	From very low to zero	Could be normal.
Mortality	0-10% (depends on initial condition)	20-40%
Dehydration	Heavy	Deep

Step 1: Begin intensive therapy

- Urgent insertion of two wide-lumen intravenous peripheral catheters for volumetric infusion therapy.

- Take blood tests for complete metabolic profile and other relevant tests.

- A central catheter should be inserted in the presence of severe hypotension, severe acidosis, impaired cardiorespiratory or renal parameters, lack of peripheral access, large need for repeated infusions.

- Infusion of 1 liter of 0.9% sodium chloride for 1 hour.

- Serum potassium levels should be >3 mEq/L before starting insulin therapy!

Step 2: Take a focused history and perform a physical exam.

Exam

- A history of insulin resistance in patients with diabetes is common and often indicates a diagnosis of DKA or HGS.

- DKA may also be the first manifestation in young people.

- A thorough physical examination helps to find the triggering cause and/or possible focus of infection, which is often the trigger of the hyperglycemic syndrome.

- A history of SGLT2 inhibitors (capaglifosine, empaglifosine or dapaglifosine) any of these can lead to euglycemic diabetic ketoacidosis due to permanent renal failure.

Step 3: Send the necessary tests to the lab

- Metabolic panel including electrolytes as well as serum magnesium and Phosphates.

- Blood urea nitrogen and plasma creatinine (may be falsely high due to the influence of the chemical analysis on ketones).

- Arterial blood gases with anion breakdown.

- General blood count with differential count.

- Urinalysis and urine ketones using a test strip.

- Serum ketones.

- Electrocardiogram, chest X-ray.

- Screening for a possible infectious cause as a trigger for a hyperglycemic state.

Treatment

1. Infusion therapy and correction of electrolyte disturbances.

2. Intravenous insulin therapy.

3. Watch for complications.

4. Treat the provoking cause.

Step 4: Infusion Therapy

- Patients with DKA and HGS usually have severe hypovolemia due to absolute or relative insulin deficiency, leading to osmotic diuresis.

- The average fluid loss during DKA and HGS is 8-10 liters. HHS can result in fluid loss exceeding 10 L. The goal is to replenish the total volume loss within 24-36 hours, with 50% of the resuscitation fluid administered during the first 8-12 hours.

- In hypotensive patients, use crystalloids to restore circulating blood volume.

- Crystalloids are the initial fluids of choice regardless of sodium level. Fluid resuscitation is started with 15-20 ml/kg/h of 0.9% sodium chloride for the first two hours.

- After the initial bolus, the rate of fluid replenishment may be reduced to 4-14 ml/kg/h. Fluid type will be determined by hemodynamic stability, sodium and urine levels.

- Semi-isotonic solution (0.45%) at a rate of approximately 250-500 ml/h if serum sodium is normal or elevated.

- In case of hyponatremia, isotonic solution is continued to be administered at the rate of 250-500 ml/h.

- In patients with HGS, comorbidities such as renal and cardiac dysfunction require more careful hemodynamic monitoring.

- Rapid correction of sodium and osmolality can lead to cerebral edema.

- Hypomagnesemia occurs in the early stages of DKA and requires correction. Monitor serum magnesium levels.

- Phosphorus depletion is common in DKA. Correction is recommended, for severe depletion (<1 mg/dL) and in patients with respiratory failure, heart failure and hemolytic anemia.

- Sodium bicarbonate infusion: metabolic acidosis improves with restoration of intravascular volume and tissue perfusion. There is a limited role for bicarbonate therapy, as it has not been shown to improve outcome in DKA. In addition, bicarbonate therapy is associated with side effects such as increased paradoxical intracellular and cerebrospinal acidosis, increased CO_2 production, adverse effects on tissue oxygenation and metabolic alkalosis after therapy.

- Bicarbonate therapy can be considered in the following situations: - when pH is constantly below 7.0; after 2-3 hours of treatment; when hypotensive shock is not amenable to rapid fluid replenishment and there is persistent severe metabolic acidosis. In the presence of severe hyperkalemia.

- Even in these circumstances, bicarbonate can only "buy time" until another treatment can correct the acidosis.

- Bicarbonate can be administered as a 100 mEq infusion for 4 hours until pH > 7.1.

Step 6: Begin intravenous insulin infusion

- Insulin therapy should be started only after water-electrolyte correction.

- Use regular (short-acting) insulin at a dose of 0.1 IU/kg body weight as a bolus dose and then 0.1 IU/kg/h as a continuous infusion or 0.14 IU/kg body weight as a continuous infusion without a bolus dose.

- When plasma glucose levels reach 11-13 mol/L, the insulin infusion rate can be reduced by 50% or to a rate of 0.02-0.05 IU/kg/h. If blood glucose levels do not decrease by 2-4 mmol/l/h, the insulin infusion rate should be doubled.

- The rate of blood glucose reduction should be less than 2-4 mmol/l/h.

- Rapid correction of blood glucose levels may lead to cell edema, mainly in children, which may lead to seizures and electrolyte disturbances (hypokalemia, hypomagnesemia and hypophosphatemia).

Step 7: Monitor the effectiveness of therapy clinically and biochemically

- The following signs indicate clinical improvement: improved well-being, decreased tachycardia and tachypnea, improved mental status, ability to eat by mouth.

The following biochemical parameters are indicative of DKA/GGS resolution: serum glucose levels below 11 mmol/L for DKA and below 13-16 mmol/L for GGS, serum bicarbonate levels above 18 mEq/L, venous pH above 7.30, serum anion gap below 12 mEq/L, decreased urine sugar, urine or serum ketones determined by the nitroprusside test are not reliable parameters since this test measures predominantly acetoacetate and acetone, whereas β-hydroxybutyrate is the predominant ketone in severe DKA that is not usually measured in the laboratory.

There may be a paradoxical increase in serum or ketone levels in the urine as patients improve due to the conversion of beta-hydroxybutyrate to acetone and acetoacetic acid. Direct assessment of beta-hydroxybutyrate. Effective plasma osmolality (excluding urea when calculating osmolality) below 315 mOsmol/kg. Delta anion gap/delta bicarbonate: to detect combined metabolic abnormalities as anionic and non-anionic hole, metabolic acidosis and metabolic alkalosis.

Step 8: Switch to subcutaneous insulin when stabilized

- Continue IV insulin until biochemical tests stabilize and the patient begins two meals a day.

- Switch to regular subcutaneous insulin with a half dose of total intravenous insulin, either as a fixed dose or sliding scale insulin according to protocol.

- The IV infusion should be stopped 2 hours after the first subcutaneous dose of insulin.

Step 9: Identify triggering factors

- Triggering factors must be identified and eliminated. Common factors include: missed insulin therapy, infections, pneumonia, sepsis, urinary tract infection, trauma, pancreatitis, myocardial infarction, pregnancy, stroke, and taking steroids.

Step 10: Continue supportive therapy

- Urinary catheter: consider for persistent hypotension, renal failure, anuria, and impaired consciousness. Observe strict asepsis during catheterization.

- Measure hemodynamics: static readings such as CVD, or dynamic readings in patients with shock. Also consider in the elderly with comorbidities, heart failure, or renal failure even in the absence of hypotension.

- Thromboembolic complications are common, so prevention of DVT should be done.

- Nasogastric tube: if consciousness is disturbed, insert a nasogastric tube to avoid aspiration of gastric contents.

- Prescribe appropriate antibiotics if infection is a possible trigger.

Hypoglycemia

A 70-year-old patient with type 2 diabetes mellitus was delivered with complaints of feeling unwell, nausea, vomiting for 2 days, sudden dizziness, sweating, palpitations, change in sensitivity. Blood glucose on a glucometer was 2.33 mmol/l. Impaired consciousness in diabetic patients is most often associated with hypoglycemia, most often caused by medications.

Symptoms of hypoglycemia are nonspecific, and it may masquerade as cardiorespiratory, neurological, or even psychiatric problems. The low threshold for checking blood sugar levels in all diabetic patients is to rule out hypoglycemia because it is a short-term treatable condition, and if left unchecked leads to severe morbidity and mortality.

Step 1: Promptly identify the clinical signs of hypoglycemia

- Signs of hypoglycemia can be autonomic, such as sweating, tremors, anxiety, palpitations, hunger, paresthesia, and tachycardia caused by sympathetic stimulation.

- They may be absent in patients with autonomic neuropathy or receiving β-blockers.

- Some patients have neuroglycopenic symptoms such as drowsiness, behavioral.

Step 2: Check blood glucose levels immediately

- Capillary sugar should be checked urgently with a bedside glucose meter. If possible, a venous glucose sample should be sent to the lab at the same time. Glucose meters at the treatment site usually overestimate glucose values in the lower range. Whenever hypoglycemia is suspected, always send blood for glucose assessment with a glucose analyzer.

- Glucose should not be delayed if it is not possible to check blood glucose levels immediately.

- If blood glucose levels are less than 3.89 mmol/L and symptoms improve with glucose administration, the patient's symptoms may be related to hypoglycemia.

Step 3: Administer intravenous glucose

- Promptly resolve hypoglycemia by administering 50 mL of 25-50% intravenous glucose.

- Check blood glucose levels after glucose infusion and repeat the injection until glucose levels exceed 3.89 mmol/L in two consecutive readings

- Begin intravenous glucose infusion 6 hours later with frequent monitoring of blood glucose levels in patients taking long-acting insulin, taking oral hypoglycemic agents, or with renal insufficiency, as they are prone to recurrent hypoglycemia.

Step 4: Consider alternative agents in specific circumstances.

- Injectable glucagon can be given at a dose of 1 mg intramuscularly or subcutaneously if venous access is not possible.

- Injectable Octreotide 25-50 mcg can be given subcutaneously or as an intravenous infusion in patients with resistant hypoglycemia induced by sulfonylurea or hypoglycemia induced by drugs such as quinine or quinidine.

Step 5: Consider triggers of hypoglycemia in diabetic patients.

- Missed meals/insufficient food intake.-Insulin overdose.

- Changes in therapy/dosage of hypoglycemic drugs or insulin.

- Simultaneous use of drugs that cause hypoglycemia.

-Presence   of   hepatic   or   renal   insufficiency.

Step 6: Consider hypoglycemia associated with other conditions (alcohol abuse, drug abuse, liver disorders).

- In the ICU, certain disorders are associated with hypoglycemia, and frequent monitoring of blood glucose levels should be performed in such patients. Hypoglycemia is more common when enteral feeding is intolerant and the patient is not transferred to parenteral nutrition.

Common causes of hypoglycemia in the intensive care unit:

Administration of oral hypoglycemic agents, sepsis (including malaria), liver failure, alcoholism, adrenal crisis (including steroid withdrawal), drugs, gatifloxacin, quinine, artesunate derivatives, pentamidine, lithium, propoxyphene.

Many patients in the ICU have an altered mental state and/or are under sedation, and a hypoglycemic episode may go unnoticed in these patients, so blood glucose monitoring is necessary for these patient groups.

Many patients in intensive care units are on intravenous insulin infusion. Discontinuation or intolerance of enteral nutrition and discontinuation of parenteral nutrition without simultaneously stopping insulin leads to hypoglycemia.

Continuous blood glucose monitoring, if available, will help detect hypoglycemia at an early stage.

Hyperglycemia is also an independent risk factor for mortality and morbidity in ICU cancer patients. Various factors contribute to hyperglycemia in the ICU. These include increased counterregulatory hormones (glucagon and cortisol), hepatic insulin resistance, glucocorticoid therapy, glucose-containing solutions, high-calorie enteral and parenteral nutrition.

Step 1: Check blood glucose levels. Check capillary glucose with a properly calibrated glucose meter at the point of care.

Caution is required when interpreting point-of-care glucose meter results in cancer patients with anemia, polycythemia, hypoperfusion, or medications that may interfere with glucose measurements. Arterial glucose (in patients with an arterial line) or venous glucose may be more accurate in patients with vasopressor shock, hypoxia, or anemia.

Treatment of the underlying disease should not be delayed while waiting for a laboratory glucose value.

Step 2: Assess glycemic risk.

- Patients should be asked about their diabetes history, current treatment, and recent blood sugar levels.

- Check HbA1c levels to evaluate blood glucose control. - Check for comorbidities such as hypertension, kidney disease, liver disease, pancreatitis, chronic obstructive airway disease, obesity, and coronary artery disease.   - Learn about your history of taking medications that cause hyperglycemia-corticosteroids, octreotide, β-adrenoblockers, thiazide diuretics, niacin, protease inhibitors, and neuroleptics.

Step 3: Determine the frequency of blood glucose measurements.

- All hemodynamically unstable patients, especially those receiving intravenous insulin infusion, should have their blood glucose levels checked every hour or even more frequently.

- As the condition stabilizes, this interval may be prolonged.- Initiate more frequent glucose monitoring if there is any change in patients' condition or diet.

Step 4: Determine target blood glucose levels.

- The current recommendation for cancer patients is to have blood glucose levels between 7.78 mmol/L and 10.00 mmol/L.

- Patients with an expected length of stay longer than 3 days will benefit from this control.

- For patients with shorter stays, there may be more liberal control of target sugar levels.

- More liberal blood sugar control is also recommended for diabetic patients.

Step 5: Determine insulin delivery route.

- All oral hypoglycemic agents and long-acting insulin should be discontinued during the first days of instability.

- Intravenous infusion of regular short-acting insulin is the method of choice in critically ill patients.

- The following groups of patients may be candidates for intermittent subcutaneous insulin administration: reduction therapy from intravenous insulin administration on an oral diet.

Step 6: Decide on an insulin delivery protocol.

The insulin protocol should be facility-specific and managed by the nurse.

- Every effort should be made to educate nurses to ensure compliance through periodic reviews.

- Dynamic insulin administration protocols, ideally computerized, that can monitor trends of higher or lower blood glucose levels and adjust insulin doses in a more desirable range.

For example, a diabetic patient with a blood sugar level of 13.89 mmol/L on admission should receive a 5 IU bolus of regular insulin followed by a 3 IU/h insulin infusion. The next blood sugar level after 1 hour is 15 mmol/L, another bolus of 5 units of regular insulin and increase the insulin infusion to 4 units/hour.

Example of an algorithm for intravenous insulin therapy in a patient in critical condition.

Random blood sugar level (mmol/l)	Bolus (U)	Infusion (units/hour)	At 1-5 units/h	At >5 units/h
8.39-11.06 mmol/l	0	2	Increase by 1 unit/h	Increase 2 units/h
11,11-13,83	3	2	Bolus 3 IU + increment 1 IU/h	Bolus 3 IU + increment 2 IU/h
13,89-16,61	5	3	Bolus 5 IU + addition 1 IU/h	Bolus 5 IU + addition 2 IU/h
16,67-19,39	8	3	Bolus 8 IU + 1 IU/h increase	Bolus 8 IU + 2 IU/h increase
19,44-22,17	10	4	Bolus 10 IU + 2 IU/h increase	Bolus 10 IU + 3 IU/h increase
22,22-24,94	10	5	Bolus 10 IU + 3 IU/h increase	Bolus 10 IU + increment 4 IU/h
>25	10	6	Bolus 10 IU + 4 IU/h increase	Bolus 10 IU + addition 4 IU/h

Target glucose level: 7.78-10 mmol/l

As another example, a diabetic patient with a blood sugar level on admission of 13, 89 mmol/L and normal renal function may be started on a scale of 2 at 4 U/h. A patient with renal insufficiency may be corrected on scale 1, and a patient without diabetes may be corrected on scale 3 or 4. The next blood glucose level check after 1 hour is 15 mmol/L, the scale should shift vertically (range 13.94-16.67) and the infusion rate increased to 6 U/h. The next blood glucose level will be 14.67 (target level7.78-10 mmol/L), the scale should shift horizontally to the right to an infusion rate of 9 units/h.

Another example of an algorithm for intravenous insulin therapy depending on the condition of the kidneys and the presence of diabetes.

RBS blood glucose level (mg/dL)	Scale 1 Kidney deficiency. (w/v-ed/h)	Scale 2 diabetes (w/v-ed/h)	Scale 3 (IV-Ed/h)	Scale 4 (IV-E/h)
<3.56	Treat as hypoglycemia	Do	Do	Do
3.56-7.78	zero	zero	zero	zero
7.79-11.1	1	2	3	4
11.2-13.89	2	4	6	8
13.90-16.76	3	6	9	12
16,77-19.44	4	8	12	16
19.45-22,22	5	10	15	20
>22,22	10	15	20	25

Patient treatment should be started on a specific scale depending on baseline sugar level and clinical scenario. On this scale, to achieve a target glucose level of 7.78-10 mmol/L, the insulin infusion rate should be shifted horizontally to the next or previous scale in the same row if the sugar remains within the range for that row. If the sugar level increases or decreases to another range, the infusion rate should shift vertically for that range in the same scale. Target RBS value: 7.78-10 mmol/L.

Step 7: Avoid hypoglycemia (blood glucose <3.89 mmol/L).

- Strict control of blood glucose levels (4.44-6.11 mmol/L) leads to episodes of hypoglycemia in cancer patients, which can adversely affect their outcome.

- The following groups of patients are more prone to hypoglycemia: renal failure, dialysis, liver failure, exhaustion, adrenal insufficiency.

Intolerance to enteral nutrition.

- Immediately stop the insulin infusion and give 50 ml of 25% intravenous glucose solution and repeat until the blood glucose level does not exceed 5 mmol/l

- Check blood glucose levels every 15 minutes and then decrease the frequency depending on clinical response.

- Ensure adequate carbohydrate and caloric intake either enterally or parenterally and avoid abrupt cessation.

Step 8: Avoid large fluctuations in glucose levels. Intensive care unit concentrations.

- Glycemic variability is expressed as the standard deviation of blood glucose levels.

- Glycemic variability is an independent predictor of mortality in a heterogeneous population of patients in intensive care.

The effectiveness of continuous or nearly continuous glucose monitoring and/or new algorithms aimed more specifically at reducing glycemic variability as well as average blood glucose levels requires further clinical studies in ICU patients before a final recommendation can be made.

Step 9: Avoid under- or over-treatment and safety concerns.

- Over- or under-treatment of hyperglycemia poses a great risk.

- Intensive care unit staff training is essential to enlist the support of those involved in the care of inpatients with hyperglycemia.

- Regular checks and technological measures should be performed to assess compliance with insulin regimens and achieving the target glucose range, preventing hypoglycemia, and minimizing glycemic variability.

Step 10. Switch to intermittent treatment once the condition has stabilized.

- Switch to subcutaneous insulin.

- Long-acting insulin should be superimposed on cessation of insulin infusion to prevent hyperglycemia.

- Short-acting intermittent insulin (either a fixed dose or on a sliding scale) must be established every six hours before feeding.

- Calculate the dosage, taking into account your diabetes history, type of diabetes, previous insulin dose, stress level, steroid use, risk of hypoglycemia, and overall clinical status.

Modern Critical Care Endocrinology, An Issue of Critical Care Clinics, 1st Edition
Author: Rinaldo Bellomo.

Hypercalcemia

Hypercalcemia is the most common metabolic disorder seen in cancer patients and is a major cause of mortality as well as morbidity. Cancers that can manifest with hypercalcemia include myeloma, lymphoma, and cancers of the lung, breast, cervix, ovaries, and kidneys.

Hypercalcemia occurs due to: bone metastases, increased parathyroid gland secretion, both primary and secondary, increased calcitriol.

Cancerous lesions release a protein related to parathyroid hormone (PTH-rP) even in the absence of bone metastases. PTH-rP behaves like parathyroid hormone (PTH). causing bone resorption and decreased calcium release from the kidneys. It has no effect on intestinal calcium absorption. Serum calcitriol levels are also not elevated. Intact parathyroid hormone (i-PTH) levels are also not elevated. I-PTH levels will be elevated in primary hyperparathyroidism and are independent of malignancy. It is very rare for a tumor to produce PTH. Bone metastases also cause the hypercalcemia seen in breast cancer metastases. However, prostate cancer, which metastasizes extensively to bone, rarely causes hypercalcemia, meaning that it is the release of cytokines that causes hypercalcemia, not direct penetration into bone.

Pneumonic "bones, stones, moans and groans" are often used to describe the nonspecific symptoms that occur, indicating skeletal pain, kidney stones, abdominal pain and altered sensitivity. Serum calcium levels above 2.6 mmol/L cause nausea, vomiting, bone pain, constipation, polydipsia, polyuria, and weakness. Neurologic symptoms such as confusion, increased somnolence, lethargy, and coma occur when levels exceed 3.5 mmol/L. Most patients will also be dehydrated.

PTH-rP measurement has not been shown to affect outcome. However, patients with PTH-rP levels above 12 mmol/L may not respond to bisphosphonates and may be more prone to develop recurrent hypercalcemia. On the other hand, serum chloride is the more available test, and hypochloremia less than 100 mEq/L confirms the diagnosis of humoral hypercalcemia. Treatment would consist of rapid rehydration and bisphosphonate therapy. Thiazides should be avoided because they interfere with renal calcium release. Oral phosphates were used previously but are no longer recommended, and intravenous (IV) phosphates are contraindicated because they increase calcium phosphate production. Calcium levels will decrease over the next 48-72 hours after taking bisphosphonates. Calcitoninis is used where a more rapid decrease is desirable (usually normocalcemia is achieved in 12-24 h). In cases with renal insufficiency or heart failure, hemodialysis may be the best way to reduce calcium levels.

The nuclear factor κB ligand receptor (RANKL) activator found on the surface of osteoclast precursors and its ligand (RANKL) secreted by lymphocytes and also found on the surface of osteoblasts and bone marrow stromal cells, stimulates differentiation of osteoclast precursors and the beginning of bone resorption. Denosumab is a humanized monoclonal antibody with high affinity and RANKLand specificity approved for the treatment of postmenopausal osteoporosis as well as for the prevention of bone metastases. It plays a potential role in the hypercalcemia of malignancies. Osteoprotegerin, a RANKL receptor-bait and inhibitor of osteoclast maturation, has also been shown to correct hypercalcemia.

Treatment of hypercalcemia

The drug	*Typical dosage*
Physiological solution	Rapid infusion of 300-500 ml/h until euvolemia. Caution in patients with heart failure
Furosemide	20-40 mg v/v every 12-24 h. Only after euvolemia.
Pamidronate	60-90 mg v/v. Adjust infusion time to creatinine clearance
Zoledronic acid	4 mg intravenously. Use with caution in patients with renal insufficiency.
Steroids: hydrocortisone or prednisolone.	Hydrocortisone: 100 mg by IV every 6 hours. Prednisolone: 60 mg orally daily.
Calcitonin	4-8 IU/kg subcutaneously or intravenously every 12 hours. Tachyphylaxis develops rapidly.
Denosumab	Under study at this time, approved only for the prevention of bone metastases

Abbreviated name: v/v, intravenously.

Hypercalcemia

Oncologic emergencies such as hypercalcemia, tumor lysis syndrome, vena cava syndrome, and spinal cord compression are sometimes seen as intercurrent problems or occur in some cancers.

Example. A 58-year-old man with metastatic renal cell cancer was admitted with lethargy, confusion, anorexia, nausea, and constipation. He had polyuria and polydipsia for the past few days.

Step 1: Resuscitation.

- Hydration is of paramount importance in these patients, and intravenous saline should be administered promptly after confirmation of hypercalcemia. Intravenous saline increases the SCF and renal excretion of calcium (Ca) ions.

Step 2: Sending and Interpreting Tests

- Measure ionized serum calcium (arterial or venous).
- If total serum calcium is being measured, make an adjustment for albumin levels. Adjusted calcium = measured total calcium + [0.8 × (4.0 - albumin)].

- Assess the severity of hypercalcemia, mild: <12 mg/dL, moderate: 12-14 mg/dL, and severe: >14 mg/dL.

- Also check serum creatinine, phosphate, and alkaline phosphatase. - Low serum chloride levels (<100 mEq/L) indicate malignant hypercalcemia.

ECG changes in hypercalcemia. ECG abnormalities reflect altered transmembrane potentials affecting conduction, such as QT interval shortening (frequent) and QRS interval prolongation (high levels). The T waves may flatten or invert, and varying degrees of heart block may develop.

Step 3: Infusion Therapy

- Severe hypercalcemia is usually associated with severe hypovolemia. - Inject 500-1000 ml of saline in the first hour and continue at a rate of 200-300 ml/h until volume replenishment and a diuresis of 100-150 ml/h is achieved.

- In patients with impaired cardiorespiratory and renal function, aggressive infusion therapy should be carried out with careful hemodynamic monitoring.

Step 4: Start diuretics after replenishing fluids

- Loop diuretics should not be used routinely.

- In patients with heart failure and/or renal insufficiency, it is reasonable to use loop diuretics to prevent volume overload.

- Consider prescribing loop diuretics only when normovolemia has been achieved, since hypovolemia causes renal hypoperfusion, preventing calcium excretion. Furosemide inhibits calcium resorption in renal tubules.

- Diuretics are especially useful if signs of hypervolemia develop, secondary to aggressive infusion therapy.

Step 5: Start specific therapy

- First-line therapy bisphosphonates, which block bone resorption by osteoclasts.

Use zoledronic acid with caution in patients with renal insufficiency and adjust the dose according to creatinine clearance.

A human monoclonal antibody, denosumab, binds to RANKL (a soluble protein necessary for the formation, function and survival of osteoclasts).

Treatment of hypercalcemia

The drug	*Dosage*	*Commentary*
Physiological solution	250-500 ml/h up to euvolemia, then 100-150 ml/hr I.V., may 3-4 L	Infusions may be required for 1-3 days depending on the patient's condition and cardiovascular and renal function. Caution in patients with congestive heart failure
Target diuresis up to 100 ml/h		
Furosemide	20-40 mg v/v	After volume correction

First-line therapy

Bisphosphonates	Pamidronate: 60-90 mg v/v for 2-24 h in 50-200 ml of normal saline (NS) Allow at least 7 days before withdrawal	Caution in renal failure May cause flu-like symptoms with fever, chills, and headache
Zoledronic acid: 4 mg w/v for 15 min in 50 ml NS		
Denosumab	120 mg subcutaneously every 4 weeks; inject an additional 120 mg on days 8 and 15 during the first month	Hypertension, fatigue, nausea, arthralgia, and hypocalcemia

Second-line therapy

Glucocorticoids	Prednisolone: 20-40 mg/day orally for 10 days	Hyperglycemia, immunosuppression
Hydrocortisone: 100 mg intravenously every 6 hours for 3 days.		
Calcitonin	4-8 IU/kg subcutaneously or v/m every 12 h	A quick start, but not a long one

Step 6: Reduce your calcium intake

- Eliminate dietary sources of calcium.

- Stop taking medications such as thiazide diuretics (increase calcium reabsorption) and vitamin D, which increase calcium levels.

Step 7: Consider dialysis

- Dialysis should be considered in patients with renal failure and/or congestive heart failure when aggressive hydration and bisphosphonates cannot be used.

Step 8: Treat the cause

- Treat the malignancy with chemotherapy and radiation therapy to control hypercalcemia if possible.

Step 9: Assess prognosis

- Patients with advanced malignancy can usually have hypercalcemia.

Hyponatremia and SIADH

Low sodium levels can occur as a result of the tumor itself or as a result of treatment. Manifestations can be simply tachycardia, irritability, and hypotension, or quite severe, such as seizures and coma. Sodium levels are an indication of intracellular volume, so high sodium levels can lead to edema; whereas low sodium levels are an indication of depleted intracellular volume. Euvolemic hyponatremia usually results from inadequate secretion of antidiuretic hormone (SIADH) syndrome and is considered a manifestation of small cell lung cancer. It can also result from chemotherapeutic agents such as cisplatin (also causes nephropathy with salt loss), cyclophosphamide, periwinkle alkaloids, ifosfamide, and imatinib. Treatment of hyponatremia consists of correction of low sodium levels. Rapid correction is not done as it may lead to myelinolysis of the bridge. Correction for sodium per L infusion = change in serum sodium (Na) in mEq/L = [(sodium infusion-Na in serum)/((weight in kg x 0.6) + 1)].

The Na content of 3% saline is 513 mEq/L and that of 0.9% saline is 154 mEq/L. SIADH is treated by limiting the amount of water administered; however, make sure that the patient does not become dehydrated. Measurement of urine and serum osmolality will help in the diagnosis and treatment of SIADH.

Example. A 67-year-old chronic smoker, diagnosed with small cell carcinoma, was hospitalized with impaired sensation, nausea, and dizziness. His vital signs were stable. Functional liver tests, urea and creatinine were normal. Serum sodium was 118 mEq/L and serum potassium was 3.0 mEq/L.

Step 1: Start the treatment

- Assess and ensure airway patency in a patient with severe hyponatremia who cannot maintain airway patency.

- The patient may need assisted ventilation.

Place a peripheral catheter and resuscitate with appropriate fluids if necessary.

- In a patient with simultaneous hypovolemia and hypoosmolality, correction of volume deficit should have priority over correction of osmolality.

- In a patient with hyponatremia, initial infusion therapy should be given with caution.

Step 2: Take a focused history and perform a physical examination.

Examine .

- This should be done to assess the severity of hyponatremia and the urgency of correction.

- Immediately pay attention to neurological symptoms such as headache, lethargy, stunting, disorientation, drowsiness, impaired consciousness, or seizures regardless of the duration of hyponatremia.

- Remember that the symptoms of hyponatremia reflect neurological dysfunction caused by cerebral edema. Cerebral edema is caused by decreased serum osmolality, which causes water to move into the cells.

- Note other symptoms of hyponatremia, such as anorexia, nausea, dizziness, and balance problems.

- Examine previous records of serum sodium levels to evaluate the chronic form.

- In chronic hyponatremia caused by cerebral adaptation, neurological symptoms are much less severe.

- Patients with chronic hyponatremia may appear asymptomatic despite a serum count below 120 mEq/L.

- Symptoms of chronic hyponatremia that may occur include nausea, fatigue, lethargy, dizziness, gait disturbances, forgetfulness, confusion, and muscle spasms.

- Seizures and coma are not usually seen in chronic hyponatremia and often reflect the acute worsening of hyponatremia.

- Ask about a history of electrolyte-rich fluid loss (prior to vomiting, diarrhea, or taking diuretics), which may indicate hypovolemia.

- Ask about a history of excessive water consumption.

- Identify a history of low protein intake and/or high fluid intake. diuretics, mannitol, desmopressin (dDAVP), intravenous immunoglobulin, and medications acting on the central nervous system, including some antidepressants, antiepileptics, and antipsychotics.

- Ask around and look for any signs and symptoms of adrenal insufficiency or hypothyroidism

- A history of hyponatremia.

- Look for a history of malignancy, HIV, liver failure, or plasma cell dyscrasia or renal failure.

- Look for signs of depleted extracellular volume, such as decreased skin turgor, low jugular vein pressure, or orthostatic/stable hypotension, which may be a consequence of hypovolemia.

- Look for signs of fluid overload, such as edema of the feet, ascites, and pleural effusion, which may be related to heart failure, cirrhosis of the liver, or renal failure. Determine the severity of symptoms - mild, moderate, or severe.

- Determine the need for hospitalization - a patient who develops acute symptoms with severe hyponatremia.

Step 3: Determine etiology

- Assess volumetric status, measure serum and urine osmolality, and measure urine sodium content.

- Whenever hyperglycemia is present, adjust the serum sodium concentration to determine the correct sodium level and rule out hypertensive hyponatremia. Remember that sodium concentration will decrease by approximately 2 mEq/L for every 100 mg/100 mL (5.5 mmol/L) increase in glucose levels.

- Patients with serum lipemic, severe mechanical jaundice, or known plasmacytic dyscrasia may have pseudohyponatremia. This laboratory artifact occurs when sodium is measured by plasma photometry.

- Find out if the patient has had recent surgery using large volumes of electrolyte-depleted solutions, irrigation fluid (e.g., adenomas or intrauterine procedures), or treatment with mannitol, glycerol, or intravenous immunoglobulin that causes isoosmolar or hyperosmolar hyponatremia.

- Assess serum creatinine concentration to determine GFR. Thiazide (or thiazide-type) diuretics, which are important causes of hypotonic hyponatremia, strongly decrease the GFR.

- In patients with hyponatremia due to heart failure or liver cirrhosis, clinically evident peripheral edema and/or ascites.

- Patients without edema with hypotonic hyponatremia have either euvolemia or hypovolemia.

- Most patients with hypovolemic hyponatremia may have obvious signs of volumetric exhaustion; however, some patients with hypovolemia may have more subtle signs and are mistakenly considered euvolemic.

- Calculate serum osmolality.

Calculation formula: Osmolarity = 2 x {Na (mmol/L) + K (mmol/L)} + glucose (mmol/L) + urea (mmol/L) + 0.03 x total protein (g/L)

Risk factors for neurological complications in hyponatremia

Acute cerebral edema	Osmotic demyelination syndrome
Postoperative patients and young women	Overly rapid correction of sodium Serum sodium less than 105 mEq/L Associated hypokalemia
Children	Undernourished patients
Patients with psychotic polydipsia	Alcoholics
Burn patients	
Older women taking thiazides	

Normal: 275-290 mOsm/kg. Serum osmolarity should always be measured rather than calculated to differentiate between hypo-, hyper-, and isoosmolar types of hyponatremia.

- Serum tonicity (effective serum osmolality) is a parameter perceived by osmoreceptors; serum tonicity controls the transcellular distribution of water. Water can freely cross almost all cell membranes and move from an area with lower tonicity (higher water content) to an area with higher tonicity (lower water content).

- The main difference between tonicity and osmolality is that tonicity reflects the concentration of dissolved substances that are difficult to penetrate through cell membranes (mainly sodium salts with a small contribution of glucose) and therefore control the movement of water between cells and extracellular fluid.

- On the other hand, osmolality also includes osmotic contributions of urea and (if present) ethanol or other alcohols or glycols, which are considered "ineffective" osmolics because they can pass and equilibrate freely through the cell membrane and therefore have little effect on water movement.

- A patient with true hyponatremia will have low serum osmolality.

- Urine osmolality less than 100 mOsm/kg: with low serum osmolality: suggests excessive water intake.

- Urine osmolality greater than 100 mOsm/kg: reflects impaired renal excretion of water (e.g., cirrhosis, prerenal renal failure) or salt (e.g., nephropathy with salt loss) or SIADH.

- Urine osmolality can be calculated from the last two digits of urine specific gravity × 30.

- Measurement of sodium concentration in urine: less than 20 mEq/L or more than 20 mEq/L.

- Measuring the concentration of sodium in the urine and assessing the volume condition will help to know the etiology.

- These parameters are not applicable in patients receiving diuretics or who have congenital kidney disease.

Step 4: assess the severity of hyponatremia

- Mild hyponatremia - 130-134 mmol/l

- Moderate hyponatremia - 120-129 mmol/l

- Severe hyponatremia - less than 120 mmol/l

Step 5: Submit additional research

In addition to serum osmolality, urine osmolality, and urine sodium, send additional tests to determine the cause and severity of hyponatremia.

- K, Cl, serum bicarbonates

- Serum glucose, urea, creatinine, total protein, triglycerides, uric acid.

- Arterial blood gases

- Serum TSH, cortisol

- Urine - creatinine, uric acid

- Fractional sodium excretion (FE Na) = (U Na × P Cr)/(P Na × U Cr) × 100.

Step 6: Correct serum sodium levels

- The treatment of hyponatremia in hospitalized patients has four goals:

✓ Prevent further decrease in serum sodium concentration.

✓ Reduce intracranial pressure in patients at risk of cerebral wedging.

✓ To relieve symptoms of hyponatremia

✓ To avoid overcorrection of hyponatremia.

Treatment of hyponatremia should be individualized.

The following factors must be considered:

✓ Severity

✓ Duration

✓ Symptoms

- The risk of complications is higher in acute hyponatremia and requires aggressive therapy.

- Chronic hyponatremia with lower serum sodium concentrations also has a greater risk of complications from overtreatment, and it needs to be monitored to avoid overcorrection.

- Patients with acute severe (i.e., serum sodium levels less than 120 mEq/L) symptomatic hyponatremia should be treated as inpatients.

- The risks of treatment (osmotic demyelination) must be balanced against the benefits. Overly rapid sodium correction is the most important risk factor for osmotic demyelination syndrome.

Step 7: Determine the rate of sodium correction

- The goal of initial therapy for severe hyponatremia is to increase serum sodium levels by 4-6 mg-eq/L within 24 hours. Thus, in the symptomatic patient achieve this within 6 hours or less, and for the rest of the time just maintain to avoid overcorrection. In symptomatic patients, sodium may be corrected at 1-2 mEq/L for the first few hours or until the seizure disappears.

In asymptomatic patients, the rate of correction should not exceed 0.5-1.00 mEq/L/h and less than 8 mEq within the first 24 h. A correction of 4-6 mEq/L
seems sufficient to avoid rapid correction.

- Avoid overcorrection of serum sodium concentration.

- Avoid isotonic solution in symptomatic hyponatremia, except in hypovolemic states with osmotic demyelination syndrome (ODS). In a patient requiring emergency treatment, sodium levels can be rapidly corrected in the first few hours of the 24-hour period.

Sodium 1 mEq = 1 mmol = 23.0 mg. 1 g = 43.5 mmol

Potassium 1 mEq = 1 mmol = 39.1 mg. 1 g = 25.6 mmol

Na+ deficiency (mmol/L) = (142 mmol/L - patient's plasma Na in mmol/L) - 0.2 body weight (kg). If correction of hypotonic dehydration is performed against a background of metabolic acidosis, sodium is administered as bicarbonate, in case of metabolic alkalosis - as chloride.

Step 8: Calculate the sodium deficit and the rate of sodium increase.

- Sodium deficiency = total body water (TBW) × (desired Na in serum - measured Na in serum).- TBW = body weight (kg) × Y.

Y =	Children	Adults men	Adults women	The Elderly men	The Elderly women
0,6	0,6	0,5	0,5	0,45	0,4

- This formula is mainly used in the reduced volume condition and in SIADH to estimate the initial fluid administration rate.

- For example, in a 60 kg woman with a serum sodium level of 115 mEq/L to increase sodium by 8 mEq/L in the first 24 hours, sodium deficiency = 240 eq.

- A three percent hypertonic solution contains approximately 500 mEq of sodium per liter, or 1 mEq per 2 ml. So, 480 mL (240 mEq of sodium) of hypertonic solution over 24 hours or 20 mL/h will increase serum sodium by 8 mEq (from 115 mEq/L to 123 mEq/L in 24 hours or 0.25 mEq/h).

- This should be confirmed by frequent serial measurements of serum sodium.

- Increased serum sodium levels with any fluid intake = (Infusion sodium - serum sodium)/Total Body Water (TBW) + 1.

- In cases where potassium is added to intravenous fluid, increase in serum sodium = [(infusion sodium + potassium) - (serum sodium)]/TBW + 1.

For example, in a 60 kg woman with a serum sodium of 110 mEq/L, if 1 L of isotonic saline (containing 154 mg-eq/L sodium), the estimated increase in serum sodium would be 4 mEq/L .

- That is, the serum sodium level will be 111.4 mEq/L after administering 1 L of saline.

- Rule of thumb - For hypertonic (3%) saline solution. Infusion rate = weight (kg) × desired correction rate. For example, to correct 1 mEq/L/h in a person weighing 50 kg- Infusion rate = 50 × 1 = 50 ml/hr.

To correct for 0.5 mEq/L/h in a person weighing 70 kg- Infusion rate = 70 × 0.5 = 35 ml/h.

- For isotonic (0.9%) saline- 0.9 NaCl is corrected at 1-2 mEq/L for every 1 L of NaCl.

- Keep in mind that these formulas are approximate, as they do not account for water translocation, main cause correction, or permanent water loss.

- Elevated sodium levels should always be confirmed by repeated sodium measurements.

- If the osmolality of the infusion fluid is less than the osmolality of the urine, paradoxically serum sodium may fall after fluid infusion.

Step 9: euvolemic, hypoosmolar, hyponatremic Consider Inadequate ADH Secretion Syndrome (SIADH)

- Clinical euvolemia.

- SIADH is the most common cause of hyponatremia in euvolemic patients with high urine osmolality.

- Diagnosed after ruling out other etiologies.

- The rate of sodium excretion is determined by sodium intake, as is normal. SIADH is often associated with hypouricaemia (serum uric acid concentration less than 4 mg/dL) due to increased urinary excretion of uric acid, and low blood urea nitrogen levels due to increased urea clearance.

- Serum sodium less than 134 mEq/L

- Urine osmolality more than 300 mOsm/kg H O_2

- Urinary sodium concentration over 40 mmol/l

- Normal kidney, liver, adrenal and thyroid function

- Serum osmolality less than 275 mOsm/kg H O_2

- In patients with severe symptoms: give 3% hypertonic solution, check serum sodium levels frequently. In patients with confusion and lethargy, initial administration of hypertonic solution to increase serum sodium levels.

The goal is to increase serum sodium levels by 1 mEq/L per hour for 3-4 hours.

Serum sodium levels should be measured after 2-3 hours and the subsequent infusion rate should be adjusted to achieve a correction rate of no more than 6-8 mEq/L during any 24-hour period.

- In asymptomatic and mildly asymptomatic patients: fluid restriction is the mainstay of treatment in most patients with SIADH, with a recommended intake of less than 800 mL/day; do not restrict fluid in subarachnoid hemorrhage, as fluid restriction may contribute to cerebral vasospasm in these patients.

Fluid restriction is defined as consumption of less fluid than is excreted with urine. Prescribe oral salts in tablets (1 g NaCl = 17 mEq). Use intravenous saline such as hypertonic saline, which should have a higher electrolyte concentration than the urine electrolyte concentration. Isotonic saline is rarely effective and often leads to a further decrease in serum sodium. Potassium is as osmotically active as sodium. Thus, giving potassium (usually with concomitant hypokalemia) can increase serum sodium concentration and osmolality in patients with hyponatremia. Intracellular sodium transfers to extracellular fluid in exchange for potassium, and extracellular chloride moves into cells along with potassium, so increasing cellular osmolality promotes free water into cells and increases sodium levels.

- If diuresis is very low and urine osmolality is low, loop diuretics can be added.

Loop diuretics, like furosemide, inhibit sodium chloride reabsorption in the thick ascending part of the Genle loop and interfere with the counterflow mechanism and cause a state of resistance to antidiuretic hormone (ADH), resulting in the production of less concentrated urine and increased water loss.

- If there are no contraindications, consider prescribing vasopressin antagonists (vaptans).

There are several receptors for vasopressin ADH: V1a, V1b and V2.

V2 receptors mainly mediate the antidiuretic response, whereas V1a and V1b receptors mainly cause vasoconstriction and mediate the release of adrenocorticotropic hormone (ACTH) respectively. The V2 receptor, Conivaptan, blocks the V2 and V1a receptors. Vasopressin receptor antagonists cause selective water diuresis (also called aquaresis) without affecting sodium and potassium excretion. The loss of free water contributes to the correction of hyponatremia. Thirst is significantly increased by taking these drugs, which may limit the increase in serum sodium. Oral tolvaptan is available and recommended for use in these patients with hyponatremia due to SIADH. Dose 15 mg once daily up to a maximum dose of 60 mg. daily - Tolvaptan should not be used longer than 1 month and should not be prescribed in patients with liver disease (including cirrhosis). Conivaptan, a V1a receptor blocker, may impair renal function in patients with cirrhosis because terlipressin, a V1a receptor agonist, has been used to treat hepatorenal syndrome.

- Demeclocycline can also be administered for SIADH at a dose of 600-1200 mg/day.

- In all cases of SIADH, eliminate the underlying cause and eliminate any medications with side effects.

Other causes of euvolemic, hypoosmolar hyponatremia such as hypothyroidism, adrenal insufficiency, renal insufficiency and psychogenic polydipsia should be treated with water restriction, hormone replacement therapy and treatment of the underlying disease.

- Hyponatremia with osmostat reset is a variant of SIADH and should be suspected in any patient with mild to moderate hyponatremia (usually between 125 and 135 mEq/L) that remains stable over time despite sodium and water balance variations. The SIADH recommendations do not apply to patients with reset osmostat (with lower osmolality ADH secretion). Treatment should primarily focus on the underlying disease (neurological conditions such as epilepsy or paraplegia).

Step 10: hypervolemia, hypoosmolarity, hyponatremia

- Consider edematous conditions such as cirrhosis, nephrotic syndrome, heart failure, and renal failure.

- Patients with hyponatremia due to heart failure or cirrhosis usually have advanced disease and present clinically with peripheral edema and/or ascites along with a previous diagnosis of heart or liver failure.

- There is no evidence yet that correction of hyponatremia improves the hemodynamic disturbances associated with severe underlying chronic heart failure or that it improves clinical outcomes.

- The main indications for specific therapy true hyponatremia are a sodium concentration below 120 mEq/L (severe hyponatremia) and/or the presence of symptoms that may be associated with hyponatremia.

In heart failure with hyponatremia, they should be treated as follows: fluid restriction, loop diuretics, angiotensin converting enzyme inhibitor (ACE) or angiotensin II receptor blocker (ARB) and loop diuretic, possibly added to increase serum sodium concentration.

Tolvaptan may play a role in the treatment of hyponatremia in patients with chronic heart failure when other treatment options have failed to raise serum sodium levels above 120 mEq/L and/or relieve symptoms of hyponatremia. Treatment of underlying disease. Avoiding additional sodium intake.

Liver cirrhosis with hyponatremia

- Withdrawal of beta-blockers, alpha-blockers, diuretics (especially thiazide diuretics).

- Correction of hypokalemia.

- Treatment of patients with persistent hypotension. Midodrine is commonly used to raise blood pressure in patients with cirrhosis. In patients with severe symptoms, try to raise serum sodium levels with an infusion of albumin and hypertonic solution.

- Hemodialysis for severe renal dysfunction.

Step 11: hypovolemic, hypoosmolar, hyponatremic

- Consider volume loss status (renal or extrarenal).

- They should be corrected as follows:

    ✓ Replenishing volume

    ✓ Treatment of the underlying disease

Low urine sodium level (<20 mEq/L). Urinary sodium less than 20 mEq/L in patients with hypovolemia caused by fluid loss from the gastrointestinal tract (e.g., diarrhea), movement of fluid into the "third space" (e.g., pancreatitis), hypovolemic hyponatremic patients with metabolic alkalosis caused by vomiting, urinary sodium concentration may be above 20 mEq/L, but urinary chloride concentration will be low (less than 20 mEq/L).

This is due to metabolic alkalosis with decreased volume and subsequent loss of bicarbonate in the urine, which negates the study of urinary sodium as a marker of hypovolemia.

High urinary sodium and chloride levels (>40 mEq/L). Sodium and chloride concentrations typically above 40 mEq/L are seen in hypovolemia and hyponatremia, in patients with renal salt loss.

Diuretic-induced hyponatremia.

- May mimic SIADH because it can be clinically euvolemic.

- Occurs mainly when taking thiazide diuretics.

- May occur within a few days of starting diuretics.

- Older patients with low body weight are more vulnerable.

- Could be due to increased water consumption.

- Treated by discontinuation of diuretics, isotonic or hypertonic solution for symptomatic

- High risk of rapid correction after discontinuation of diuretics.

- Close monitoring is required to avoid osmotic demyelination.

- Patients with hyponatremia who exhibit clinical symptoms and signs of hypovolemia may have extrarenal fluid loss or renal fluid loss.

- Measurement of urine. Sodium and chloride concentrations can often make a difference. - Patients without edema with hypotonic hyponatremia have either euvolemia or euvolemia.

 - Sometimes both SIADH and thiazide-induced hyponatremia may be present because of the underlying disease and the diuretic used, respectively.

Cerebral salt depletion (CSW)

- This can mimic SIADH because the laboratory findings are similar.

- Hyponatremia with low plasma osmolality.

- Unreasonably high urine osmolality (> 100 mOsm/kg and usually > 300 mOsm/kg).

- Urinary sodium concentration above 40 mEq/L.

- Much rarer than SIADH.

- It occurs in acute CNS lesions, mainly with subarachnoid hemorrhage.

- Clinically hypovolemic.

 - Normal serum uric acid level.

- Increased fractional excretion of urate.

- This can be distinguished from SNSADG.

Treatment

- Treat underlying causes of CSW, such as subarachnoid hemorrhage.

 - Place a central catheter to assess volume status.

 - Replenishment of the volume that corresponds to the loss of urine.

 - Required amount of sodium = sodium deficiency × total amount of water in the body.

 - Blood products if anemia is present.

Step 12: Hyperosmolar hyponatremia

 - Consider hypertonic mannitol, glycine or other osmotic agents and hyperglycemia.

The difference between SIADH and CSW

	CSW	SIADH
Plasma volume	Decreased	Normal or elevated
Salt balance	Negative	Plain
H_2O balance	Negative	Increased or unchanged
Signs of dehydration	available at	Absent
Body weight	Decreasing	Increased or unchanged
WDC	Decreasing	Elevated or normal
Hematocrit	Increased	Elevated or normal
AMK/creatinine ratio	Increased	Plain
Serum protein concentration	Enlarged	Plain
Potassium concentration in serum	Increased or unchanged	Reduced or no change
Serum uric acid concentration	The usual	Decreasing

PKVP - pulmonary capillary congestion *pressure*, CVP - central venous pressure, AMI - blood urea.

Patients with recent prostate or uterine surgery. Absorption of non-conductive glycine, sorbitol, or mannitol solutions for irrigation during prostate or bladder TUR or during hysteroscopy or laparoscopic surgery may decrease serum sodium levels by increasing extracellular fluid volume with these sodium-free solutions.

- Treatment: Stop the infusion. Correction of hyperglycemia: stop or reduce glucose infusion. Administer insulin and fluids. Bring blood glucose concentration to 4.7-8 mmol/L.

Step 13: Isoosmolar hyponatremia

- Rule out pseudohyponatremia (improper blood draw, hyperlipidemia, paraproteinemia, plasma cell dyscrasia, and patients with mechanical jaundice).

- Usually asymptomatic.

- No treatment is required.

Literature

Critical Care Medicine: An Algorithmic Approach, 1st Edition
Author : Alexander Goldfarb-Rumyantzev 2023.

Modern Critical Care Endocrinology, An Issue of Critical Care Clinics, 1st Edition
Author : Rinaldo Bellomo 2019.

TUMOR LYSIS SYNDROME (TLS)

As the name implies, these emergency conditions result from tumor death, sometimes spontaneous, but usually as a result of ongoing chemotherapy. Commonly seen in high tumor mass, acute lymphoblastic leukemia, acute myeloid leukemia, Burkitt's lymphoma, small cell lung cancer, germ cell tumors, breast cancer, melanoma.

Metastases to the liver may also increase the risk of tumor lysis syndrome (TLS). In some patients with chronic lymphocytic leukemia treated with fludarabine or 2-chlorodeoxyadenosine, this syndrome may occur even 2 weeks after treatment.

Tumor lysis syndrome (TLS) results from the release of intracellular ions during cell death, resulting in hyperkalemia, hyperphosphatemia, and elevated theuric acid levels. There is secondary hypocalcemia as a product of calcium phosphate is formed. Symptoms are usually manifested by lethargy, irritability, seizures, decreased diures or anuria or arrhythmias. This is confirmed by laboratory findings of hyperkalemia, hyperphosphatemia, elevated uric acid levels, and renal dysfunction. The Cairo-Bishop classification is used for diagnosis. Treatment usually includes increasing the amount of renal lavage fluid, ensuring no additional potassium in intravenous fluids, and no prescribed potassium-saving drugs, diuretics, if there are volume overload features. Allopurinol, Kidney. There is currently no role for alkalinizing urine. Rasburicase, or recombinant uratoxidase, is an enzyme that has a protective effect on the kidneys and can be used.

Laboratory determination of tumor lysis syndrome using the Cairo-Bishop classification.

- Uric acid>8 mg/dL or 25% increase from baseline

- Potassium > 6 mEq/L or 25% increase from baseline

- Phosphorus> 6.5 mg/dL or 25% increase from baseline baseline

- Calcium <7 mg/dL or 25% reduction from baseline- Clinical tumor lysis syndrome

- Creatinine level> 1.5 times the upper limit of normal

- Cardiac arrhythmia or sudden death

- Seizures.

Note: Two or more laboratory changes should be observed within 3 days before or 7 days after chemotherapy.

Treatment of metabolic disorders in tumor lysis syndrome

Problem	*Care*
Hyperphosphatemia	Minimize consumption with restrictions on dairy products and bread

Phosphate binders (aluminum hydroxide or aluminum carbonate) 30 ml every 6 h in adults	
Dialysis if there is no response to oral therapy	
Hyperkalemia	Insulin 10 IU IV with 50 mL 50% dextrose IV, then administer 50-75 mL of 5% dextrose for one hour
Albuterol inhalation	
Diuretics such as furosemide	
Dialysis if there is no answer	
Hypercalcemia	Use with caution in the presence of hyperphosphatemia. If the patient is symptomatic, intravenous calcium gluconate
Hyperuricemia	Allopurinol 100 mg/m2 orally every 8 hours (maximum daily dose: 800 mg)
Rasburicase 0.15-0.2 mg/kg/day v/v 2nd dose may be based on observed response	
Renal failure and hypovolemia	Intravenous administration of saline solution, 3 L/m^2 per day. Use with caution in reduced systolic function
Dialysis for oliguric renal failure unresponsive to fluid administration or in patients with CHF	

Abbreviations: IV, intravenous, CHF, chronic heart failure, where rapid reduction of uric acid and
the presence of renal damage.

Rasburicase is not administered to pregnant women or patients with glucose-6-deficient phosphate dehydrogenase (G6PD). If there is anuria, then dialysis may be required. Dyselectrolycemia requires treatment as well as insulin and glucose, diuretics and potassium binders for hyperkalemia, phosphate binders for hyperphosphatemia, but hypocalcemia is not corrected if the patient has no symptoms.

Clinical example. A 26-year-old patient with Burkitt's lymphoma recently started chemotherapy. The clinical presentation is anorexia, lethargy, disorientation, vomiting, muscle cramps, tachypnea, and decreased diuresis.

Step 1: Intensive therapy

- These patients are usually dehydrated and will benefit from intravenous fluids

Step 2: Get a diagnosis

- Tests may reveal hyperuricemia, hyperkalemia, hyperphosphatemia, hypocalcemia, uremia, and elevated lactate dehydrogenase levels.
Get an electrocardiogram to rule out serious arrhythmias and conduction disorders.

- Tumor lysis is associated with malignancies such as acute lymphoblastic leukemia or Burkitt's lymphoma with a high tumor mass, and these tumors respond quickly to chemotherapy.

- Usually follows chemotherapy, but can occur after radiation, corticosteroid therapy or chemoembolization and rarely spontaneously.

- Check diuresis and kidney function.

- Factors associated with the patient's tumor can be used to assess the risk of SLO.

Step 3: Start infusion therapy

This strategy is useful as a preventive measure in patients at high risk for SLOs and in patients with established SLOs.

- A high fluid infusion rate is appropriate.

- Patients at high risk for tumor lysis syndrome should have aggressive volume as a preventive measure before chemotherapy.

- Pour isotonic fluid at a rate of 200-300 ml/h.

- The volume should be adapted to the patient's age, cardiac function, and diuresis.

- Increasing the rate of urine flow is the most effective strategy for preventing obstructive uropathy induced by urate.

- Diuresis should be maintained between 80-100 ml/h (4-6 ml/kg/h).

- Urine specific gravity should be maintained at ≤1.010.

Step 4: Use diuretics with caution

- Maintain adequate diuresis.

- Contraindicated in the presence of hypovolemia or obstructive uropathy.

Step 5: Alkalizing the urine

- Not currently recommended specifically for patients with elevated phosphate levels.

- This can lead to the formation of xanthine crystals in the urine, which can cause renal tubular obstruction if allopurinol is used at the same time.

- Urine alkalization is not recommended for the prevention and therapy of SLOs

Step 6: Prescribe allopurinol

This should be considered in patients at intermediate risk of SLO and pre-treatment with uric acid levels < 8 mg/dL.

- Purine catabolism leads to the formation of hypoxanthine and xanthine, which are metabolized to uric acid through the enzymatic action of xanthine oxidase.

- This pathway can be blocked with allopurinol, a hypoxanthine analog that competitively inhibits xanthine oxidase.

- Start allopurinol orally at 600 mg/day if uric acid is below 8 mg/dL.

- Allopurinol should be started at least 24 hours before chemotherapy.

- After about 2-3 days of allopurinol therapy, increased excretion of hypoxanthine, which is more soluble than uric acid, and xanthine, which is less soluble than uric acid, is noted.

- A marked increase in xanthine excretion can occur when allopurinol is prescribed to prevent tumor lysis syndrome and can lead to acute renal failure or xanthine stones.

- It should be used with caution in patients with renal insufficiency, may cause skin hypersensitivity reactions.

- Allopurinol should be prescribed only in patients at low to moderate risk for TLS. Additional treatment options should be considered if TLS is established.

- Febuxostat can be used if the patient is hypersensitive to allopurinol.

Step 7: Consider rasburicase (recombinant ura toxidase)

This should be considered in patients at high risk for SLOs and in patients with impaired heart or kidney function and pre-treatment uric acid levels > 8 mg/dL.

- Uratoxidase - present in most mammals but not in humans - oxidizes pre-formed uric acid to allantoin, which is five to ten times more soluble than uric acid.

- When administering exogenous uratoxidase (uricase, rasburicase) the uric acid level in the urine decreases markedly within about 4 hours.

- This should be used especially if the uric acid level is above 8 mg/dL.

- Uric acid levels should be monitored regularly to adjust the dosage.

- Rasburicase degrades uric acid in blood samples at room temperature, thus interfering with accurate measurement.

- Therefore, the samples should be immediately placed on ice until the analysis is completed.

- Rasburicase should not be administered to patients with G6PD deficiency because of the risk of severe hemolysis.

- If rasburicase administration is needed in an emergency and G6PD results are not immediately available, it can be administered at a low dose of 0.02-0.05 mg/kg, with provision for urgent dialysis in cases of hemolysis.

Step 8: Treat concomitant electrolyte disturbances

- Hyperkalemia - hemodialysis may be necessary if renal failure is present or volume overload is present.

- Hypocalcemia - if it is asymptomatic, no therapy is needed.

- Hyperphosphatemia - limit phosphate intake and increase loss with phosphate-binding agents such as aluminum hydroxide or calcium carbonate, sevelamer hydroxide and lanthanum carbonate.

Step 9: Consider hemodialysis

- This method should be considered in certain situations, such as:

- Volume overload

- Uric acid level more than 10 mg/dL, despite rasburicase

- Uncontrolled hyperkalemia and hyperphosphatemia

- Calcium X phosphate ratio >70

- Renal failure

The above discussion is not exhaustive, but serves as a guide to bring these patients to the attention of the treating physician.

Rapid Response Events in the Critically Ill, 1st Edition A Case-Based Approach to Inpatient Medical Emergencies Editors : Arsalan Zaidi & Kainat Saleem

Textbook of Critical Care, 7th Edition Editors : Mitchell P. Fink & Jean-Louis Vincent & Frederick A. Moore.

Delirium in adult cancer patients: ESMO clinical guidelines.

Delirium is a neurocognitive syndrome that usually occurs in the elderly and in people with cancer, especially in those with advanced disease and in the last hours or days of life. While the underlying malignancy and its complications predispose a person to developing delirium, many of the treatments used to treat cancer also increase the risk of delirium.

Risk factors for delirium are often described as "predisposing" or "triggering. "Predisposing" factors refer to those conditions that already exist in the individual at baseline and increase
susceptibility of a person to the development of delirium, while the "provocative"
factors are those responsible for the activation of a particular episode delirium. Because delirium is ubiquitous, it is possible that people who have had cancer without active disease, but who have developed cognitive impairment as a result of cancer exposure and/or treatment, may also be at risk for developing delirium.

Direct risk factors for delirium. Factors associated with cancer:

- Primary CNS tumors
- Secondary CNS tumors
- metastases to the brain - meningeal metastases
- Paraneoplastic neurological syndromes

Toxicity of antitumor treatment. Brain irradiation: acute or delayed encephalopathy. Chemotherapy: methotrexate, cisplatin, vincristine, procarbazine, asparaginase, cytarabine (cytosinarabinoside), 5-fluorouracil, ifosfamide, tamoxifen (rare), etoposide (high doses), nitrourea compounds, alkylating agents (high doses or arterial route)

Indirect risk factors for delirium

Metabolic encephalopathy due to hepatic, renal or pulmonary insufficiency. Electrolyte disorders, including SIADH. Disorders of glucose levels. Infections, sepsis - any localization, including intravenous injections. Hematologic disorders. Nutritional deficiencies (Thiamine (vitamin B1, Folic acid (vitamin B 9, Cobalamin (vitamin B_{12}) , dehydration; non-convulsive status epilepticus, vasculitis, Medications (anxiolytics, sleeping pills, opioids, corticosteroids, NSAIDs, Anticonvulsants, Anticholinergic agents, Scopolamine (hyoscine hydrobromide), Atropine, belladonna alkaloids, Drugs with established anticholinergic activity, such as tricyclic antidepressants, diphenhydramine, promethazine, trihexyphenidyl, hyoscine butyl bromide.

Other psychoactive substances: neuroleptics, antidepressants, levodopa, lithium. Anti-infectives: ciprofloxacin, acyclovir, ganciclovir. Histamine H blockers$_2$. Omeprazole. Immunomodulators: interferon, interleukins, cyclosporine. Medication polypragmasy. Other status or predisposing comorbidities: age> 70 years, pre-existing cognitive impairment such as dementia, history of delirium, hearing impairment.

Indirect risk factors for delirium

Other status or predisposing comorbidities. Visual impairment. Urinary retention or use of a urinary catheter. Constipation Alcohol or drug abuse or withdrawal (including nicotine) CNS disease or injury; history of stroke or transient ischemia; liver failure. Renal failure.

Terminal stage of heart disease. Terminal stage of lung disease. Endocrinopathy.

The standardized Cochrane Risk Alert Study focused on three categories of medications: opioids, dose>80 mg parenteral equivalent of morphine daily; benzodiazepines, dose 2 mg equivalent of lorazepam daily; and taking anticholinergic agents, corticosteroids, and anticonvulsants.

Prevention recommendations:

• Given the lack of studies evaluating pharmacologic prophylaxis of delirium in cancer patients, no evidence-based recommendations are offered. Physicians should also avoid inappropriate prescribing. For prevention, avoidance of risk factors is recommended.

Treatment recommendations:

-Opioid rationing (or switching) to fentanyl or methadone is an effective strategy in the context of opioid-associated delirium.

-The standard approach to opioid-associated delirium in clinical practice is to reduce the dose or switch to another opioid (with a 30-50% reduction in the dose of the opioid equianalgesic.

-Prescribing neither haloperidol nor risperidone is of obvious benefit in the symptomatic treatment of mild to moderate delirium and is not recommended in this context.

-In clinical practice, it can be difficult to clearly classify delirium as mild or moderate. Because haloperidol and risperidone are ineffective in cancer patients with mild to moderate delirium and have been shown to worsen symptoms, it can be argued that these drugs are also likely to be of no benefit and may be harmful in delirium classified as severe. Further trials of neuroleptics are needed to confirm this.

-The administration of olanzapine may be useful in the symptomatic treatment of delirium. The administration of quetiapine may be useful in the symptomatic treatment of delirium. Administration of aripiprazole may be useful in the symptomatic treatment of delirium. Quetiapine is available in oral forms only for acute care, whereas olanzapine and aripiprazole are also available in parenteral or oral forms, but use with caution because of the long elimination period. Sedation is a well-known side effect of olanzapine and quetiapine, which may have an advantage in patients with hyperactive delirium.

• Methylphenidate can improve cognitive function in hypoactive delirium, in which there is no delirium or perceptual disturbances and the cause is not identified.

-Benzodiazepines are effective in providing sedation and,

possibly anxiolysis in the emergency treatment of severe symptomatic distress associated with delirium. Although midazolam and other benzodiazepines are very widely used in palliative care for many reasons, they are not considered part of the initial treatment strategy for delirium. The clinical decision to use midazolam or lorazepam in the treatment of delirium (especially in patients with agitation and regardless of whether they are already taking antipsychotic medications) should include an assessment of the patient's level of distress; safety risks with and without benzodiazepines; and patient mobility. Nevertheless, benzodiazepines play a first-line role in the treatment of alcohol or benzodiazepine withdrawal.

Delirium is usually refractory in the antemortem phase. If restless agitation associated with delirium persists, pharmacological sedation in the last hours, days or 1-2 weeks of life may be required in the form of palliative sedation.

Delirium in adult cancer patients: ESMO Clinical Practice Guidelines. Annals of Oncology 29 (Supplement 4): iv143-iv165, 2018 doi:10.1093/annonc/mdy147.

CHAPTER 4 SUPPORTIVE THERAPY FOR CANCER COMPLICATIONS

Cancer Pain

Cancer-related discomfort is experienced by most people who have been diagnosed. Some people experience chronic discomfort even after completing therapy. Effective pain management is necessary to preserve the quality of life of cancer patients and requires an accurate diagnosis. The treatment of pain in cancer is very challenging because of the vast differences in patients' responses to different treatments and medications. Studies show that heredity can affect opioid sensitivity; consequently, opioid doses can vary greatly from person to person. Consequently, it is very important *to individualize* treatment, taking into account the diverse pharmacology of opioids and the varying drug susceptibility of individuals. Accurate classification of pain makes it possible to determine its origin and mechanism, thus determining the choice of treatment. Identifying modulators of pain severity, such as psychological distress, alcoholism, substance abuse and delirium, allows physicians to more accurately tailor therapeutic recommendations.

Breakthrough cancer pain (BCP) is a subtype of cancer pain characterized by short-term exacerbation of pain in patients with stable baseline background pain. It is formally defined by a rapid onset (within minutes), high intensity, and pain aggravation that lasts more than 30 minutes. Given its heterogeneity, it has proven to be a complex pain condition that is difficult to treat. Understanding both pain-related and patient-associated conditions is crucial to treatment, which is highly individualized.

The two main mechanisms of pain are **nociceptive** (somatic or visceral) and **neuropathic**.

Nociceptive pain results from irritation of pain receptors and **neuropathic** pain from direct involvement of the peripheral nervous system or CNS.

Somatic pain usually occurs with bone metastases, musculoskeletal pain, inflammation or after surgery and is well localized, dull or aching pain.

Visceral pain results from infiltration and compression by tumor or bloating of internal organs and is described as a diffuse, deep, squeezing, pressure sensation.

Neuropathic pain is caused by tumor infiltration of the peripheral nerves, roots, or spinal cord, as well as chemical damage caused by chemotherapy, radiation therapy, or surgery. This pain is described as sharp or burning.

These three types of pain can occur individually or in combination. Adult cancer pain can be divided into three levels based on a numerical scale of 0-10: mild pain (1-3), moderate pain (4-6), and severe pain (7-10).

Pain control in patients whose antitumor therapy options have been exhausted. Life expectancy in such patients, as a rule, does not exceed 2-6 months. In these cases, the main method of pain control is the administration of opioids.

Basic principles of pain control:

The analgesic medication must be administered noninvasively (i.e., no injections). The oral route is the most preferable, transdermal or transmucosal administration of drugs is possible. Of the parenteral routes of administration, the subcutaneous route is considered the main route, and if there is a need for rapid pain control (e.g., in a severe attack), the intravenous route is the main route. **Intramuscular route** for permanent pain relief **is**

not used. Epidural and intrathecal administration of opioid analgesics may be used in some patients with severe pain and poor response to conventional systemic opioid therapy.

2.   The analgesic drug should be administered regularly, at regular intervals, taking into account the elimination half-life (i.e. "on the clock"), without waiting for the pain to get worse.

3.   Doses are adjusted as follows: from high doses of weak opioids to low doses of strong opioids.

4.   The analgesic medication is selected individually, taking into account the patient's characteristics and reactions. Pain control is achieved by selecting an adequate dose (titration) of the opioid to provide pain relief until the next dose is administered.

5.   The effectiveness of therapy should be evaluated regularly, anticonvulsants and antidepressants should be used to control neuropathic pain, and adjuvant, or adjuvant drugs (ion pump blockers, corticosteroids, antispasmodics, benzodiazepines, antihistamines, local anesthetics) and side effects should be used.

Basic recommendations for pharmacotherapy of pain:

Pain management for cancer is usually treated with a stepwise approach (i.e., the "WHO Ladder"), depending on the level of pain.

Step 1: Patients with mild pain who are not taking opioids can begin treatment with non-opioid analgesics, including NSAIDs or acetaminophen. First stage of pharmacotherapy: mild pain (0-4 HRS score). Hepato- and nephrotoxicity inherent to non-opioid analgesics, as well as gastro-toxicity and cardiovascular risks inherent to NSAIDs, should be considered when choosing a drug.

Step 2: Patients with no response to neopioids or with moderate pain are treated with weak opioids such as codeine, hydrocodone and oxycodone alone or in combination with acetaminophen.   Step 2: Moderate pain

(4-7 points). Neopioid analgesics are ineffective. Opioids + non-opioid analgesics ± adjuvant drugs are recommended. Weak opioids (tramadol) are used, in some cases low doses of strong opioids.

Step 3: Severe pain is treated with opioids such as morphine, hydromorphone, methadone, or transdermal fentanyl. Tramadol, which has a weak affinity for μ-opioid receptors and is considered a non-opioid medication, can be used in patients with mild to moderate pain that does not respond to NSAIDs and those who wish to delay opioid treatment. Co-analgesics should be prescribed in individual cases. Stage 3: severe pain (7-10 points) that is not adequately controlled by regular administration of stage 2 drugs and adjuvants. Strong opioid analgesics are recommended; if necessary, prescribe additional non-opioid analgesics and adjuvant drugs.

Systemic *corticosteroids* may be helpful for pain caused by metastatic bone lesions, increased intracranial pressure, spinal cord compression, compression, or nerve infiltration.

Tricyclic *antidepressants* such as nortriptyline and anticonvulsants such as gabapentin are usually indicated for neuropathic pain. Bisphosphonates (zoledronic acid and pamidronate) and radioactively labeled substances (strontium-89 and samarium-153) can help treat pain associated with bone metastases.

Common side effects of opioid therapy include constipation, nausea, respiratory depression and sedation. Constipation should be prevented with prophylactic use of combined laxatives and stool-promoting softeners. If symptoms persist, patients may be helped by supplementation including lactulose, magnesium citrate, polyethylene glycol, or enemas. Patients who experience inadequate pain relief despite aggressive opioid therapy or who cannot tolerate opioid titration because of side effects may benefit from interventional therapy such as regional infusion of analgesics and neuroablative or neurostimulatory procedures.

Uncontrolled pain should be considered a medical emergency. Patients in acute pain may often require opioid administration through a patient-controlled dose. These patients require close monitoring. Bone metastases are commonly seen in patients with prostate, breast, lung, kidney, and bladder and myeloma cancers.

Bone scans (nuclear imaging with technetium-99m) are sensitive to blast lesions but not to lytic lesions). As for bone scan lesions, they should be evaluated with conventional radiographs or CT scans to identify lesions at risk for pathological fractures.

Pain should be controlled aggressively with opioids. NSAIDs may offer additional relief. Lesions at risk of fracture should be treated surgically or with radiation therapy. Bisphosphonates and RANK ligand inhibitors may reduce fracture risk and pain.

Consider options for combining the different groups to reduce the dose and side effects of the drug when used alone.

Multimodal pain management protocols include a PLANNED (regular, hourly!) prescription of NSAIDs and a PLANNED prescription of paracetamol.

The WHO is constantly conducting information campaigns to make it clear to patients and doctors that intramuscular injections almost never have an advantage over other ways of administering drugs!

Switch to oral analgesics as soon as possible!

For example, paracetamol 650-1000 mg orally (!) every 6 hours scheduled(!), ibuprofen 600 mg orally (!) every 6 hours scheduled(!) after intravenous ketorolac 15-30 mg for breakthrough pain or other NSAIDs.

Thus, it is important for effective pain relief:

- Denial of anesthesia "at the patient's request"!

- Observance of intervals:

~ 6 h for Neopioid Analgesics

~ 4 h for Morphinomimetics

!!Регулярное (from часам!!) the administration of analgesics is important to limit the need for opioid analgesia for breakthrough pain.

Histone deacetylase inhibitors (HDACs) are being studied in clinical trials for their ability to increase the effectiveness of chemotherapy. Animal studies show that some HDAC inhibitors can prevent and reverse CIPN (Cancer Induced Peripheral Neuropathy)

Opioids, nonsteroidal anti-inflammatory drugs (NSAIDs), acetaminophen, antidepressants, anticonvulsants, NMDA antagonists, and alpha-2-agonists are commonly recognized pharmacological treatments for cancer.

Side effects associated with existing pharmacological treatments for cancer pain.

Opioids: sedation, dizziness, nausea, vomiting, constipation, physical dependence, tolerance, and respiratory depression.

NSAIDs: poor digestion, stomach ulcers, headaches, drowsiness, dizziness, gas, bloating, heartburn, nausea, vomiting

Acetaminophen: nausea, stomach pain, loss of appetite, itchy rash, headache, dark urine, clayey stools.

Antidepressants: headache, nausea, dry mouth, insomnia, dizziness, diarrhea or constipation, sexual problems, fatigue

Anticonvulsants: dizziness, drowsiness, fatigue, nausea, tremor, rash, weight gain.

N-methyl-D-aspartate (NMDA) *antagonists*: hallucinations, dizziness, vertigo, fatigue, headache, out-of-body sensations, nightmares, sensory changes.

Alpha-2 agonists: depression, bradycardia, orthostatic hypotension, constipation, nausea, upset stomach, dry mouth.

New pharmacological effects of cancer pain treatment

Celina G. Virgen, Pharmacological Management of Cancer Pain: Novel therapeutics, 2022., Tapentadol is a centrally acting analgesic with two synergistic modes of action because it binds to the MOR opioid receptor and inhibits noradrenaline reuptake (NRI).

TCelecoxib/Parecoxib, a selective COX-2 inhibitor, is used to treat cancer pain and has fewer gastrointestinal side effects than non-selective NSAIDs.

Duloxetine is a serotonin and norepinephrine reuptake inhibitor approved for many indications, including severe diabetic neuropathy, and plays a role in the treatment of neuropathic pain in part by inhibiting P2X receptors activated on microglia.

Tetrodotoxin (TTX) is a powerful neurotoxin mainly found in puffins. It inhibits sodium channels, which play an important role in the transmission of pain signals. One article evaluated the role of TTX in bone cancer pain.

Botulinum toxin type A (BTX) BoNT-A is a strong neurotoxin produced by Clostridium botulinum that prevents the release of acetylcholine at the presynaptic level in muscle tissue, thereby blocking the action potential in the neuromuscular junction. BoNT-A potential as an analgesic drug for both nociceptive and neuropathic cancer pain.

TRPM8 Receptor activation on cooling in neuropathic pain models suggested a unique target for cooling-induced analgesia /Data from preclinical studies show that activation of the transient receptor potential melastatin 8 (TRPM8) ion channel by topically acting drugs causes significant analgesia

Growth factor inhibitors. Recent clinical and preclinical studies have linked the epidermal growth factor receptor signaling pathway to chronic pain conditions.

Lemairamine (agonist of α7 nicotinic acetylcholine receptors (α7nAChRs)) Lemairamine (wgx-50) is extracted from the pericarp of the plant Zanthoxylum. It can reduce neuroinflammation in Alzheimer's disease as an agonist of the 7 nicotinic acetylcholine receptors (7nAChRs).

Denosumab (Prolia) is a type of targeted therapy called a monoclonal antibody. It is the first drug approved to treat bone pain caused by metastatic cancer and bisphosphonates such as alendronate (Fosamax) and is considered a first-line therapy for bone pain caused by cancer.

PAR2 receptor protease 2 (PAR2)-activated *antagonists* are being studied for the treatment of pain in oral cancer.

Tanezumab is another potential new treatment for bone pain caused by metastatic cancer. Tanezumab is an antibody that blocks the activity of a pain-signaling molecule called nerve growth factor (NGF).

Recommended reading

1.	Celina G. Virgen, Neil Kelkar, Aaron Tran, Christina M. Rosa, Diana Cruz-Topete, Shripa Amatya, Elyse M. Cornett, Ivan Urits, Omar Viswanath, Alan David Kaye, Pharmacological man-agement of cancer pain: Novel therapeutics, Biomedicine & Pharmacotherapy, Volume 156, 2022, 113871, ISSN 0753-3322, https://doi.org/10.1016/j.biopha.2022.113871.

2.	Management of cancer pain in adult patients: ESMO Clinical Practice Guidelines. Annals of Oncology 29 (Supplement 4): iv166-iv191, 2018. doi:10.1093/annonc/mdy152.

3.	Gruzdev V.E., Anisimov M.A. Multimodal continuous approach to pain management in oncological patients (clinic's first experience). MD-Onco 2022;2(1):33-8. (In Russ.). DOI: 10.17650/2782-3202-2022-2-1-33-38.

Application of adjuvant therapy (multimodal analgesia strategy, low-opioid analgesia, etc.)

Consider using a multimodal pain management strategy, which may be the key to improved treatment outcomes.

Approximate scheme can be applied when the intensity of the pain syndrome is more than 5 points on the HACS.

Basis therapy is based on oral administration of drugs (paracetamol in a dose of 1 g 3-4 times a day intravenously (not more than 3 days, in the absence of contraindications), and then - oral administration of gabapentin 300 mg 3 times a day and celecoxib 200 mg 2 times a day. This combination provides a multimodal effect while minimizing side effects.

In severe pain syndrome with a tonic muscular component, the combined drug neodolpasse (75 mg diclofenac and 30 mg orphenadrine) is prescribed in a dose of 250 ml intravenously 2 times a day instead of celecoxib. In the presence of significant cardiovascular disease - naproxen 150 mg 2 times a day. Of antidepressants, either zoloft 25 mg or mirtazapine 15 mg daily is prescribed. If there is no effect and breakthrough pain, consider an elastomeric pump with a formulation including the powerful and manageable opioid fentanyl. Nefopam, which is a non-narcotic, centrally acting analgesic, is used to enhance its effect and reduce the dose of the narcotic analgesic. It has practically no side effects (except tachycardia when administered intravenously by jet injection). When patients have contraindications to NSAIDs, it replaces them in combination with paracetamol. Can be used in patients with terminal stage of chronic renal failure, provided that the single and daily doses are reduced twice

To correct side effects of fentanyl and nefopam (nausea and vomiting), ondansetron, a central selective blocker of serotonin 5-HT3 -receptors, is included in the mixture. Approximate base case (fentanyl 800 mcg, nefopan 100 mcg, ondansetron 24 mg + sodium chloride 0.9% 100 ml at 2-8 ml/hr, i.e. 16-64 mcg/hr for fentanyl). Consider using other forms of fentanyl as transdermal forms (nasal, bucal) or tramadol in a base pump, adding ketamine using large volume pumps (300 or 600 ml). The dose of ketamine is administered at a subnarcotic analgesic dose of 0.25-0.3 mg/kg/h.

Do not forget about lidocaine, which prevents the development of secondary hyperalgesia caused by the formation of excessive Na+-channels in the area of damaged tissues. It activates the descending inhibitory system, including by enhancing the release of endogenous opiates.

Consider switching to "opioid-free" pump formulations when managing breakthrough pain: lidocaine - no more than 1.5 mg/kg/h (maximum daily dose 2000 mg), ketamine - no more than 0.3 mg/kg/h, (dissociative doses >1 mg/kg/h), nefopam - no more than 120 mg/day (maximum daily dose), dexmedetomidine - no more than 0.2 µg/kg/h. Note that components may not be used because of side effects for a particular patient, for example: nonsteroidal anti-inflammatory drugs for thrombocytopenia or acute ulcer, nefopam for marked tachycardia and nausea, dexmedetomidine for bradycardia and hypotension, somnolence, etc.

Gruzdev V.E., Anisimov M.A. Multimodal continuous approach to pain management in oncological patients (clinic's first experience). MD-Onco 2022;2(1):33-8. (In Russ.). DOI: 10.17650/2782-3202-2022-2-1-33-38.

Fatigue

A common symptom in cancer, occurring in about 80% of patients with advanced disease. Close attention should be paid to any signs of underlying depression, which should be managed appropriately.

Fatigue may be due to:

- cancer treatment, including chemotherapy, radiotherapy, surgery, and some biological therapies:
- different cancer treatments can affect your energy level in different ways, the type and schedule of treatment can also affect the degree of fatigue caused by cancer treatment;
- taking medication for nausea (a feeling of impending vomiting) and painkillers;
- The accumulation of toxic substances as the cancer affects the cells;
- lesion of normal cells;
- by an increase in temperature (above 100.4 °F or 38 °C);
- infection; pain; dehydration; loss of appetite or not getting enough calories and nutrients; sleep problems; anemia; shortness of breath; less active lifestyle; other illnesses.

Care

The first step in treatment is to identify treatable comorbidities such as pain, poor nutrition, emotional stress, sleep disturbance, and comorbidities (anemia, infections). Appropriate pain management, nutritional support, sleep therapy, exercise, and necessary supportive care can help address some of these issues. Transfusion support and erythropoietin may be helpful in anemic patients. Psychostimulants such as **methylphenidate** or **modafinil** may be helpful in some patients with severe symptoms.

Anorexia and cachexia

Anorexia is defined as loss of appetite associated with weight loss.

Cachexia is a metabolic syndrome characterized by profound involuntary weight loss.

Choosing cachexia treatment options: prioritization and multimodal care.

Given the complex and multifaceted mechanism of cachexia, treatment of cachexia should be based on a comprehensive assessment of the patient and an evaluation of reasonable available treatment options, food intake may be impaired by many factors and secondary to the symptoms of nutritional effects, some of which may be treatable. If, after addressing these factors, food intake is still inadequate, nutrition-based interventions should be initiated.

Compared with providing energy and nutrients through nutritional interventions, modulating metabolic disturbances is more complex. The development of insulin resistance and also anabolic resistance impair the maintenance of total muscle mass. Thus, interventions to reduce catabolism and enhance anabolic pathways include providing adequate energy and protein; muscle training; pharmacological agents to increase appetite, reduce systemic inflammation, and stimulate muscle growth; and psychosocial interactions to alleviate stress.

When antitumor treatment is offered to a patient with cachexia, the intensity of multimodal supportive treatment, including nutrition, exercise, anti-catabolic and anti-inflammatory treatment, and psychological and social support, must be monitored in addition to careful dosage adjustments. In cachexic cancer, nutritional support and physical therapy may be offered on an individual basis, with careful monitoring of individual goals and quality of life.

In patients undergoing anti-cancer therapy and/or with an expected survival of at least several months, adequate energy and nutrient intake should be adhered to. Nutritional support in patients who are able to eat should be based on dietary recommendations, recommendations for high calorie, high protein foods, food fortification (e.g., adding fats/oil, protein powder) and the use of oral nutritional supplements. If this proves insufficient and the lower gastrointestinal tract is working, feeding via tube should be considered or otherwise PP is the method of choice. Very few trials have compared different regimens or amounts of nutritional support. In one study that randomized patients with severely compromised food intake and a limited survival of 1-4 months, PP did not improve quality of life or survival, but it did increase the number of side effects. Similarly, another study randomizing patients showed only that PP had no effect on median survival.

Nutritional requirements. The goal of nutritional support is to ensure adequate intake of energy and nutrients, allowing the patient to eat, enjoy food, and participate as part of social life. Indications for nutritional support during chemotherapy and radiation treatment:

- BMI less than 20 kg/m^2
- loss of more than 5% of body weight in 6 months;
- hypoproteinemia less than 60 g/l or hypoalbuminemia less than 30 g/l;
- Inability to eat adequately by mouth;
- moderate to severe enteropathy.

The daily protein content should be 1-1.5 g/kg, with CKD - no more 1-1.2 g/kg, energy supply 20-30 kcal/kg. At rest, energy expenditure may increase in cachexia, total energy expenditure is often normal (25-30 kcal/kg body weight/day) due to a corresponding decrease in physical activity, but may be unpredictably low or high in some patients. Even increased energy and protein intake may not be able to attenuate weight loss in all patients. Given the presence of anabolic resistance in the elderly, protein (at least 1.2 and possibly up to 2 g/kg body weight/day) may be necessary to balance protein synthesis.

Fat utilization in weight-loss cancer patients is very high and can cover most of the energy expenditure at rest, whereas carbohydrate utilization is impaired in the presence of systemic inflammation and insulin resistance. In addition, fats have a high energy density, allowing smaller amounts to be supplied. Compared to a standard diet, an iso-azotic, isocaloric, ketogenic, low-carb diet maintains nitrogen balance and protein metabolic rate in the body. In a randomized controlled trial (RCT) conducted in cancer patients suffering from exhaustion, a high-fat diet improved weight control compared to a standard diet.

In cancer cachexia, omega-3 fatty acids have been studied, especially because of their anti-inflammatory properties in specialized ONS, usually also enriched with protein (N3P-ONS). Several randomized trials have been published on the effects of N3P-ONS on cancer patients. No adverse effects from the supplements were seen, showing benefits of N3P-ONS in patients receiving radiation therapy, chemotherapy or chemoradiotherapy. However, when administered to patients not receiving anticancer therapy, no benefit from N3P-ONS was found.

Probe feeding. Dysphagia due to obstruction, motor dysfunction, or mucosal inflammation may compromise or interfere with normal food intake and thus is an indication for tube feeding. Patients with head and neck or upper gastrointestinal cancers are at particular risk of dysphagia due to obstructive tumors, and also have severe mucositis caused by aggressive treatment (e.g., combination therapy). It is critical to recognize the onset of dysphagia in time and to respond in a timely and individualized manner to ensure adequate nutrition. Probe feeding can be associated with potentially serious complications, including mechanical (e.g., tube blockage), gastrointestinal (e.g., diarrhea), infectious (e.g., aspiration pneumonia) and metabolic (e.g., feeding resumption syndrome). Short-term RCTs have shown that the metabolic efficacy and complication rates of enteral feeding and PP are similar. Because the enteral route is more physiologic, safer, and less expensive, it is a better option if there is no serious GI dysfunction. In some conditions, supplemental PP is preferable to tube feeding; for example, if patients suffer from nausea, vomiting, abdominal discomfort, or severe diarrhea. Rather, the decision to initiate PP should be made on an individual basis, depending on the degree of illness, the patient's physical and psychological resources, and on an individual risk/benefit assessment. PP carries the risk of potentially serious complications, including (but not limited to) catheter-associated infection, blockage and thrombosis, electrolyte disturbances, feeding resumption syndrome, excicosis, fluid overload, and chronic hepatopathy and osteopathy. The authors observed improvements in fat-free mass and quality of life in favor of additional PP after 12 weeks, but saw no difference in 6-month survival.

Parenteral nutrition is indicated if adequate EP for more than 3 days is not possible.

The duration of PP:

- 10-15 days (short-term): acute and severe mucositis, ileus, uncut vomiting;

- more than 30 days (prolonged): severe malabsorption, subacute or chronic radiation enteritis, severe enteropathy against the background of "graft versus host" reaction.

Mixed nutrition (EP + PP) can be prescribed to patients simultaneously if one of these methods is not effective enough to provide more than 60% of their energy needs.

The effectiveness of the NP is monitored once every 5-7 days:

- total serum protein;

- serum albumin;

- hemoglobin;

- peripheral blood lymphocytes;

- body weight and BMI once every 7-10 days.

Under professional guidance, moderate exercise is safe for patients with cancer cachexia and is recommended for maintaining and increasing muscle mass. Weight-bearing exercises also two to three times a week, moderate aerobic exercise (endurance) should be offered to all patients with cachexia. Prescribing exercises should involve a physical therapist or properly trained professional and include a structured approach that includes modes (aerobic, resistance, flexibility), frequency, intensity and duration, as well as specific times for evaluation.

Pharmacological remedies

Several drugs have been investigated for their potential use in treating or alleviating the effects of cancer cachexia. However, only corticosteroids and progestins have consistently had beneficial effects on appetite and/or body weight (BMW), albeit at the expense of significant side effects, while for other agents, the data are patchy or disappointing.

Corticosteroids

Corticosteroids include several drugs with different glucocorticoid, mineralocorticoid, and anti-inflammatory activities. Prednisolone, methylprednisolone, and dexamethasone are the most commonly used. Symptomatic relief seems to be mainly achieved by their potent anti-inflammatory activity. Toxicity is usually negligible when used for only a few weeks, whereas with prolonged use corticosteroids can cause rapid loss of muscle mass, insulin resistance, and an increased chance of infections, such as candida and stomatitis, contributing to the deterioration of cachectic patients. Corticosteroids are recommended to control fatigue associated with cancer. Several RCTs examining the effects of corticosteroids on appetite in patients with advanced cancer. Most trials reported temporary improvements in appetite and well-being, while there was no effect on body weight or survival. The anti-anorectic effect of corticosteroids is transient and often disappears after a few weeks. There is limited data to recommend one corticosteroid over another.

Progestins

Medroxyprogesterone acetate and megestrol acetate (MA) have been widely studied for the treatment of weight loss and anorexia in cancer patients. In preclinical models, progestins stimulate appetite and inhibit the synthesis of proinflammatory cytokines. A Cochrane review including 23 RCTs on AF use in cancer patients (median duration 8 weeks) found significant improvements in appetite (relative risk 2.57) and weight gain (relative risk 1.55). However, no lasting improvement in quality of life was observed, and no data on muscle mass were available.In the studies analyzed, AF was used at doses of 160-800 mg/day and weight improvement was higher for doses >160 mg/day, while no dose effect on appetite was observed.

Treatment with AF is associated with an increased risk of thromboembolism, fluid retention, adrenal insufficiency, and hypogonadism in men. Although the aforementioned Cochrane review reported that MA does not increase the incidence of adverse events or death.

Cannabinoids

Cannabis sativa is a medicinal plant that contains several cannabinoids, including tetrahydrocannabinol (THC). Medicinal cannabis is available in a variety of forms, such as tablets/capsules, vaporizer, or mouth spray. In patients with cancer cachexia in small trial and case series studies, THC appeared to improve appetite and slow weight loss. However, larger randomized trials found no significant effect on appetite or quality of life; toxicity was low in these trials.

Androgens. In cancer patients, hypogonadism is associated with progressive cancer status, weight loss, and most likely opioid use. Anabolic androgenic steroids have been shown to reduce loss of muscle mass and strength in patients with wasting associated with acquired immunodeficiency syndrome. The use of androgens has not been studied intensively in patients with cancer cachexia. In an RCT of 37 lung cancer patients, a nandrolone analog did not improve muscle mass compared to placebo. In a three-group RCT including 496 patients with cachexia, fluoxymesterone at a dose of 10 mg twice daily was significantly inferior to MA at a dose of 800 mg/day to improve appetite.

Olanzapine

Olanzapine is an atypical antipsychotic that acts on multiple receptors, including dopamine and serotonin receptors, both of which are potentially associated with cachexia. In clinical use, olanzapine causes an increase in body weight and an increase in appetite compared to other antipsychotics. In a recent RCT, olanzapine significantly reduced nausea not caused by chemotherapy in 30 patients with advanced cancer compared with placebo. Thus, olanzapine may be considered for the treatment of chronic nausea in patients with advanced cancer.

Nonsteroidal anti-inflammatory drugs

Nonsteroidal anti-inflammatory drugs (NSAIDs) block cyclooxygenase pathways and reduce inflammation by inhibiting prostaglandin production. NSAIDs have been studied to reduce the catabolic urge for systemic inflammation in patients with advanced cancer and cachexia. In a systematic review including six controlled trials and seven observational trials, 11 of these trials reported an increase or stabilization of MT or fat-free body weight with little report of side effects. The body of evidence, however, was weak. Thus, in cachectic patients in need of pain control, NSAIDs may be considered with potential additional benefit in improving MT.

Prokinetics

Metoclopramide and domperidone are widely used for treatment of early satiety, chronic nausea, and dyspepsia and gastroparesis. However, no large RCTs have investigated the role of prokinetics in cachexia. While one RCT in patients with advanced cancer showed that metoclopramide can reduce nausea but not appetite, no similar studies have been conducted with domperidone. Metoclopramide and domperidone can cause serious, mostly neurological, side effects, such as tardive dyskinesia, cramps, depression, dizziness, and urinary retention.

Ghrelin receptor agonists

Anamorelin has recently been approved in Japan for the treatment of cancer cachexia in patients with non-small cell lung cancer, gastric cancer, pancreatic cancer and colorectal cancer, but it is not approved in Europe based on findings from the ROMANO trial showing a more modest improvement in muscle mass compared to that observed in the Japanese trial.

Combination therapy.

Published trials focusing on potential synergism between pharmacologic agents such as progestins, antioxidants, L-carnitine, thalidomide, n-3 fatty acids, and NSAIDs have been unsuccessful or unreliable because of methodological flaws.

Recommendations

Corticosteroids can be used to increase appetite, but with a short period of up to 2-3 weeks. The effect on appetite usually disappears with longer treatment. Progestins can be used to increase appetite and MT, but not muscle mass, quality of life, or physical function in patients with cancer cachexia. The risk of serious side effects, including thromboembolic events, must be considered. There is insufficient evidence to support the use of medical cannabis or its derivatives to alleviate anorexia in patients with cancer cachexia. Because there is no evidence of a lack of beneficial effects in terms of improving muscle mass, androgens are not recommended. There is moderate evidence to suggest the use of olanzapine to treat appetite and nausea in patients with advanced cancer. There is insufficient evidence to recommend the use of NSAIDs alone to treat cancer cachexia. There is insufficient evidence to recommend the use of metoclopramide or domperidone alone for the treatment of cancer cachexia.

Insufficient evidence to recommend specific combination regimens because of the lack of evidence from large, well-designed randomized trials. Patients may benefit from pharmacologic therapy in addition to caloric supplementation. Megestrol acetate is active, with symptomatic improvement in less than 1 week.

Despite a rapid increase in appetite, it may take several weeks to achieve weight gain. Megestrol is also associated with an increased risk of thromboembolism and should be used with caution. Dexamethasone provides short-term improvement, usually without significant weight gain. Dronabinol has limited benefits for anorexia and is associated with sedation.

Recommended literature.

Cancer cachexia in adult patients: ESMO Clinical Practice Guidelines

https://www.esmoopen.com/article/S2059-7029(21)00049-1/fulltext#secsectitle0125

Hemotransfusion practices and complications.

In oncology, about 40% of patients receive hemotransfusions and blood transfusions are common practice. It is usually safe, but can sometimes lead to minor or life-threatening consequences if one is not attentive to details and protocols.

Step 1: Therapy

- Attach two large diameter cannulas (14G/16G) for intravenous infusions.

- Send blood for blood typing, cross-matching, complete blood count (CBC), coagulation profile, and other relevant tests.

- In these situations, proper coordination with the blood bank is mandatory. for early and correct blood products.

Step 2: Transfer red blood cell mass or blood components

If the patient is bleeding profusely and hemodynamically unstable, consider a "universal donor" blood transfusion pending blood compatibility.

- In hemodynamically stable patients cross-matched blood for a particular group is used. There are no advantages of using fresh blood over old blood.

- If there is active bleeding, transfuse quickly within 30 minutes (if possible, use a rapid infusion pump that can administer fluids at a higher rate).

- 4 ml/kg of red blood cell mass (usually one unit) increases hemoglobin by 1 g/dL and hematocrit by 3% in the absence of active bleeding.

Alternative methods of reducing complications for red blood cell mass

Leukoreduction. Purpose: to minimize the risk of cytomegalovirus transmission, reduces febrile nonhemolytic transfusion reaction and alloimmunization. Indications: high risk in immunocompromised patients who require multiple transfusions, patients who have had febrile nonhemolytic transfusion reactions, recurrent severe allergic reactions despite premedication, IgA deficient patients, patients at risk of hyperkalemia, transfusions to relatives. Does not prevent TA-RTPH (graft versus host reaction)

Using a certain type of filter for red blood cells and platelets during transfusion.

Washed red blood cells. Purpose: to prevent an allergic reaction. Indications: recurrent severe allergic reaction despite premedication, IgA deficient patients, patients at risk of hyperkalemia, reduction of risk of hyperkalemia, reduction of antibodies to IgA. Not equivalent leukoreduction, loss of 15-20% of red blood cells.

Erythrocytes washed with physiological solution to remove> 98% plasma, proteins, antibodies, leukocytes, and electrolytes.

Gamma irradiation to inactivate white blood cells. Purpose: prevents TA-RTPX. For infusion in premature infants, malignancy patients, allogeneic hematopoietic transplant recipients, blood transfusion to relatives. Does not reduce infection risks or FNHTR (Febrile Non-Hemolytic Transfusion Reactions).

Frozen red blood cells. Whole blood. Purpose: for persons with rare blood type, in massive blood transfusions, in weakened patients at risk of CMV infection.

Blood components and antifibrinolytics

SPP (fresh frozen plasma). All clotting factors and plasma proteins. Indications: Deficiencies and consumption of clotting factors. Dose15 ml/kg. Must be group-specific. 15 ml/kg SPP will increase clotting factors by 25-30%, which is sufficient for adequate clotting.

Thawed plasma can be stored (1-6 °C) for up to 5 days. Factor VI inversion and effect of factor V anticoagulants (warfarin). Indications: plasmapheresis replacement, elevated INR and planned invasive procedure.

Thawed plasma must be transfused within 24 hours if stored at room temperature.

Massive blood transfusion (>1 blood volume within a few hours). Use blood filters.

Cryoprecipitate. Contents: fibrinogen VIII/vWF (Willebrand factor), factor XIII, and fibronectin. Indications: for decreased fibrinogen, liver disease, post-thrombolysis, bleeding. Dose: 1 pc/7-10 kg. Must be transfused within 6 hours of thawing. 1 unit of cryoprecipitate/10 kg body weight increases plasma fibrinogen levels by ~50 mg/dL.

Platelet mass. Composition: donor platelets - approximately 8.0 thousand/mm^3 with 50 ml of plasma. Indications: bleeding due to critically reduced circulating platelets or functionally abnormal platelets. Infusion 30-60 min. Must be group-specific. Expected platelet count increase of ~7,000-10,000/mm^3 after polydonor platelet concentrate or 30,000-60,000/mm^3 for each SDP (single donor).

Single-donor platelets - 3.5-4.0 thousand/mm3 with 250 ml of plasma. Indication: when platelet count> 10,000/mm^3 in stable without bleeding, >30,000/mm^3 in unstable and >50,000/mm^3 in patients who have had invasive procedures or active bleeding> 100,000/mm^3 or in CNS trauma. A dose of 5-10 ml/kg platelets (RDP or SDP) should result in a 50-100,000/mm^3 increase.

Desmopressin. Stimulates endothelial release of factor VIII and vWF (V2 receptor-mediated effect), where they form a complex with platelets and increase their ability to aggregate. Indications: hemophilia A, Willebrand's disease, uremia, thrombocytopathy, in trauma orthopedic surgery, liver transplantation, bleeding during prostatectomy. The dose of 0.3 µg/kg is repeated until clinical improvement.

Activated factor VIIa. Composition: activated protein C. Indications: Factor VIIa deficiency. Dose: 30 to 90 µg/kg, repeated every 2 to 3 hours until satisfactory hemostasis. Tachyphylaxis may occur after three to four doses and 12-24 h intervals are necessary.

Antifibrinolytic drugs.

Tranexamic acid action competitive inhibitor of plasminogen activation. Bolus dose 10-15 mg/kg intravenously then 1 mg/kg/h for 5-8 h.

Epsilon aminocaproic acid. Competitive inhibitor of plasminogen activation. Indications: hyperfibrinolysis, operations requiring artificial circulation, liver transplantation and some urological and orthopedic surgeries. 100 mg/kg as an intravenous bolus followed by an infusion of 15 mg/kg/h (maximum 24 g/day).

Aprotinin. It is a polyvalent inhibitor of proteolytic enzymes (trypsin, chymotrypsin, plasmin and kallikrein). which leads to inhibition of fibrinolysis, inhibits the contact phase of blood coagulation activation, which is a trigger factor of coagulation process and stimulation of fibrinolysis. Aprotinin is used during surgeries under conditions of artificial circulation, orthopedic surgeries, liver transplantation, reducing inflammatory reactions, leads to decreased need for allogeneic blood transfusion and reduced blood loss. It is administered by IV drip in dose of 100 000-200 000 UIC, and if necessary - up to 500 000 UIC depending on the intensity of bleeding. For prophylactic purpose in surgery, it is administered by IV or IV drip in dose of 200 000-400 000 UIC before, during and after surgery, and then by 100 000 UIC during next 2 days. Contraindications DIC, hypersensitivity to aprotinin.

Blood should be transfused within 4 hours, except in emergencies. The rate of transfusion can be adjusted as needed, i.e., rapidly in patients with hypovolemia and slowly in stable patients; however, after dispensing from the blood bank, transfusion must be completed within 4 hours to prevent microorganism growth. If the blood cannot be transfused within this time, it is recommended that it be disposed of.

- Transfuse blood and blood products through a filter sufficient to prevent the passage of small clots that may form in stored blood.

- A filter with a pore size of 170-200 μm is recommended for routine transfusions of red blood cells, platelets, fresh frozen plasma (FFP) and cryoprecipitate.

- Filters with smaller pore sizes are more effective, but they can increase resistance and filter out platelet aggregates, reducing the effectiveness of transfused platelets.

- Microaggregate filters 20-40 μm in size are recommended only for artificial blood circulation.

- Filters can reduce the transfusion rate. Therefore, the standard recommendation is to use a new set for each transfusion. For rapid transfusions, if the filter does not appear clogged, change the set every two transfusions.

- Use a blood transfusion heater for massive blood loss. This helps prevent hypothermia, which can contribute to coagulopathy by causing reversible platelet dysfunction, altered coagulation kinetics, and increased fibrinolysis.

- Hypothermia also causes ventricular arrhythmias and citrate toxicity due to decreased citrate metabolism.

- Do not use unconventional and uncontrolled methods, such as storing near heat sources or immersing the bag in a hot water bath.

Step 3: Correct coagulopathy

- Correct high INR with SPP or low platelet counts with platelet transfusions alone in a patient with active bleeding.

- Do not correct elevated INR prophylactically in a patient without bleeding unless surgical intervention is contemplated.

- Other coagulopathic disorders need to be corrected.

- Antifibrinolytic drugs can be used to minimize bleeding in situations such as trauma.

- Correct the hypothermia.

- Normalize calcium levels.

- In some specific situations, consider factor VII activation. Use rotational thromboelastometry (ROTEM) if possible to further guide transfusion strategy.

Step 4: Control the source of the bleeding

- Perform an investigation to determine the source of the bleeding and consider available treatment options (interventional radiology or surgery). - Urgent consultation with these specialties is required if necessary.

Step 5: Assess the severity of bleeding

- Massive blood loss can be defined as: loss of one blood volume within 24 hours, blood loss equivalent to 7% of fat-free body weight in an adult (5 L) and 8-9% in a child, loss of 50% of blood volume within 3 hours, blood loss at a rate greater than 150 ml/min.

Step 6: Manage massive blood loss

- Establish continuous invasive pressure monitoring for infusion therapy if the patient continues to be hypotensive due to ongoing bleeding.

- General blood count (Hb and platelets) and coagulation tests (prothrombin time, ACTV, fibrinogen), blood gas analysis, serum electrolytes (Na, K, Mg, ionized calcium) and serum lactate should be performed.

- They should be repeated frequently for ongoing bleeding and after each component of therapy.

- Transfusion of platelets, SPP, and cryoprecipitation should be guided by the results of laboratory tests.

- The administration of SPP should be started after the loss of one blood volume and platelets after the loss of 1.5 times the blood volume.

- A 1:1:2 ratio of red blood cell mass, SPP, and platelets from a random donor should be maintained to prevent dilutional coagulopathy and dilutional thrombocytopenia due to massive transfusions, which leads to a vicious bleeding cycle.

- Prescribe cryoprecipitate if fibrinogen is less than 100 mg/dL or if there is a threat
of volume overload with CPS.

- If patients with blood type A or B have received multiple units of O, rhesus-positive whole blood, they can be switched back to their group blood after testing at the blood bank.

Step 7: Identification and Treatment of Complications Caused by Transfusion

- Stop transfusion immediately if an acute hemolytic transfusion reaction occurs.

- Hypotension can be associated with acute ongoing bleeding, acute severe transfusion reaction, allergic reaction/anaphylaxis, or rarely due to septic shock (due to transfusion of blood with bacterial contamination).

- Check the recipient's last name against the information on the bag.

Transfusion-related complications

Febrile nonhemolytic transfusion reaction. Reaction between recipient antibodies and transfused leukocytes with release of pyrogenic cytokines. Clinical signs: fever, rise in temperature. Treatment: give paracetamol and resume transfusion at a slow pace.

Allergic reaction. Reaction to soluble allergens in donor plasma with development of urticaria and pruritus. Give 10 mg intravenous chlorphenamine (pheniramine maleate) or another antihistamine.

Anaphylaxis. IgA-deficient patients react to IgA during transfusion with the development of anaphylaxis (pruritus, laryngospasm, bronchospasm). Stop transfusion immediately. Insufflate O2, subcutaneous/injection 0.5 mg adrenaline, 100 mg IV hydrocortisone, 10 mg IV chlorpheniramine maleate, inhaled salbutamol, intravenous crystalloids, return blood to blood bank along with patient blood sample, use washed red blood cells in future.

Sepsis. Bacterial contamination. Clinically: fever, chills, hypotension

Stop transfusion. Gram staining and blood culture if bacterial contamination is suspected. O2, intravenous infusion, and vasopressors to maintain mean arterial pressure >65 mm Hg. Broad spectrum antibiotics if sepsis is suspected.

Acute hemolytic transfusion reaction (<24 h). It is almost always intravascular hemolysis due to immune (AB0 blood group incompatibility, or other antigenic systems or nonimmune mechanism (thermal, osmotic and mechanical injury to red blood cells in the blood component). Classical OGR includes a triad of symptoms: fever, back pain, and the appearance of red or brown urine.

Other symptoms of acute hemolysis may also be present: chills, hypotension, renal failure, back pain, or signs of disseminated blood clotting. In practice, when analyzing a large number of clinical cases, the most common, 80%, and often the only symptom that appears with erythrocyte destruction is fever or chills. Renal failure develops in only 36% of cases of acute hemolysis. The timing of symptoms can vary from a few minutes from the start of the transfusion to 24 hours afterwards. Laboratory signs of hemolysis: appearance of altered forms of erythrocytes (spherocytes), presence of free hemoglobin in blood plasma and its red staining, hemoglobinuria; reduced levels of fibrinogen and haptoglobin in blood and, conversely, increased levels of lactate dehydrogenase and bilirubin in blood. Send blood for general blood count, coagulation, Coombs direct test, lactate dehydrogenase, haptoglobin, liver function tests for indirect bilirubinemia, peripheral smear for signs of hemolysis.

Delayed hemolytic transfusion reaction (24 hours to 28 days) Delayed hemolytic reaction (DH) is due to an anamnestic immune system response to allogeneic antigens from previous transfusions or after pregnancy. The erythrocyte breakdown is mostly extravascular and clinically less dramatic. Symptoms in the form of jaundice and subfebrile fever are usually present. The laboratory changes may be identical to those of acute HG and in blood tests are: anemia, high lactate dehydrogenase (LDH) and bilirubin levels and low haptoglobin levels, leukocytosis, presence of anti-erythrocyte antibodies in the blood and positive Coombs test.

ABO incompatibility. Transfusions of incompatible blood, IgM antibody against major red blood cell antigen leading to intravascular hemolysis, renal problems, disseminated intravascular coagulation (DIC). Clinical signs: fever, chills, chest or lower back pain, hypotension, and shortness of breath. Stop transfusion. Notify the blood bank and return the blood to the blood bank. Infusion of saline solution to maintain diuresis at 100 ml/hour. Give diuretics if diuresis decreases. Treat DIC with appropriate blood components.

Transfusion-associated graft-versus-host disease is a complication of blood component transfusions as a result of immunological conflict. It is a rare complication with a very high mortality rate of 0.01 cases per 100,000 transfusions. This syndrome is caused by activation of T-lymphocytes of the transplant (blood component) with production of cytokines in the recipient that stimulate the antigenic response. Patients at highest risk of this complication are immunocompromised people receiving chemotherapy. Treatment: There is no specific treatment. Immunosuppression with corticosteroids and cytotoxic agents may help to some extent. Prophylaxis: irradiation of blood components such as red blood cells, platelets, and granulocytes. Avoid haploidentical transfusions, e.g. from close relatives.

Transfusion-related *circulatory overload* (TACO) is circulatory overload following a transfusion of blood or blood products.

- Transfusion-associated acute lung injury (TRALI) is defined as new acute lung injury (with hypoxemia and bilateral infiltrates on chest X-ray but no evidence of left atrial hypertension) occurring during or within 6 hours after transfusion, with a clear temporal relationship to transfusion and not explained as another risk factor for acute lung injury.

- Transfusion-associated *hyperkalemia* is increased in massive trauma, renal failure, and newborns/infants

- Increased risk of citrate toxicity in massive transfusions in patients with liver disease

Step 8: Use fewer allergenic blood products

- In patients with multiple transfusions and transfusion-related complications, consider using alternatively processed blood products .

Step 9: Consider the threshold for transfusion

- If bleeding has stopped and there are no clinical signs of hypoperfusion, do not transfuse any more blood or blood products.

- Maintain a transfusion threshold of less than 7.0 g/dL and 7-8 g/dL Hb in critically ill patients with stable hemodynamics in the absence of active bleeding.

- If there is active bleeding, maintain a higher transfusion threshold of 9-10 g% and be guided by clinical needs.

- Adult critically ill therapeutic and surgical patients with suspected sepsis and septic shock, a higher transfusion threshold of 8-10 g/dL may be considered during the first 6 hours of resuscitation.

- The transfusion threshold should be individualized according to the patient's hemoglobin level before hospitalization, age, hemodynamic stability, cardiac status, and availability of the appropriate blood group.

- Red blood cell transfusion may be useful in patients with anemia and acute coronary syndrome (hemoglobin level > 9 g/dL).

- Blood for patients who have undergone cardiovascular or orthopedic surgery blood transfusions to maintain hemoglobin levels of 7-8 g/dL.

- All red blood cell transfusions in stable patients without bleeding should be ordered with one unit. Check post-transfusion hemoglobin before ordering additional units.

Step 10. Use blood products judiciously

- In the absence of bleeding, do not correct a high INR with SPP.

- Patients receiving inadequate intake or taking broad-spectrum anticoagulants and antibiotics are likely to have vitamin K deficiency, which can lead to INR abnormalities.

- They benefit from intravenous vitamin K

- Consider judicious use of intravenous iron and erythropoietin where indicated to minimize the need for blood transfusions.

Step 11: Follow the transfusion protocol

- Obtain informed consent, patient identification, visual inspection of blood for hemolysis

- Use only 0.9% saline or albumin, ABO-compatible plasma through the same intravenous catheter. Initial infusion rate of 1-2 ml/min for the first 15 minutes to detect any signs of hemolytic or allergic reaction.

- Blood transfusion for no more than 4 hours.

- If necessary, hemoglobin after transfusion can be checked as early as 15 minutes after transfusion.

A 48-year-old woman with a mitral valve prosthesis on warfarin presented to the department with severe vaginal bleeding in the past 12 hours, she is pale, with cold peripheral skin, a frequent thready pulse, and tachypnoea. Her hemoglobin is 5.0 g% and her INR is 7.5.

Perform step 1 and step 2 similarly to the first case.

Step 3.

- Administer 5-10 mg of vitamin K intravenously for 15-20 minutes, which will reverse the effects of warfarin, after 4-6 h, or use prothrombin complex NWP/cryo/4 factor (PCK) concentrate to treat uncontrolled bleeding. Monitor INR for 6-8 hr.

- For less severe bleeding, oral vitamin K at a dose of 1-2.5 mg may be considered, which will lower the INR after 8-24 h.

- If there is life-threatening bleeding or bleeding in critical areas (CNS, pericardium, or airway), temporarily withdraw the anticoagulant and correct the coagulopathy with SPP/cryoprecipitate or 4-factor prothrombin complex concentrate (4F-PCC).

Various anticoagulants and their antidotes

Unfractionated heparin Laboratory tests: activated partial thromboplastin time (ATTB) IV protamine 1 mg/100 IU heparin.

Low molecular weight heparin (LMWH) laboratory test Anti-Factor Xa levels treatment IV protamine 1 mg/100 units dalteparin/tinzaparin or protamine 1 mg/1 mg dose of enoxaparin received in the previous 8 h. Consider rFVIIa for critical bleeding.

Vit K antagonist (warfarin) test: Prothrombin time (PT)/International normalized ratio (INR).

If INR <4.5 and no bleeding - do not take warfarin until INR reaches the therapeutic range. Cancel - give vit K 2.5 mg orally.

If 4.5-10 and no bleeding - discontinue warfarin, consider giving vitamin K 2.5 mg orally. Give vitamin K 2.5 mg orally or 1 mg intravenously.

If INR >10, give vitamin K 2.5 mg orally or 1-2 mg intravenously for 30 minutes.

Repeat every 24 hours. Vitamin K 1-2 mg intravenously for 30 min, repeat every 6-24 h.

Direct thrombin inhibitors: Dabigatran TT - diluted thrombin time ECT-Ecarin clotting time ECA-Ecarin chromogenic assay. If the above tests are not available then thrombin time, ACTV.

Treatment. IV idarucizumab or IV 4PCC/(aPCC) 50 units/kg, SPP is irrelevant. Anticoagulant discontinuation. Antifibrinolytic agent (tranexamic acid). Consider activated charcoal if the drug has been ingested within 2-4 hours.

Oral factor Xa inhibitors rivaroxaban, epixaban, endoxaban. Test: anti-Factor Xa levels, Normal BHTV does not exclude elevated drug levels. AChTV is not sensitive to epixaban. Andexanet alfa at 50 U/kg, discontinuation of anticoagulant, antifibrinolytic agent (tranexamic acid) Consider activated carbon if drug was ingested within 2-4 hours. Without the role of SPP.

Thrombocytopenia

A 50-year-old patient was admitted with a diagnosis of pancreatic tumor. Blood tests showed Hb of 10.7 g%, white blood cells 12,000/mm3, and platelets 110,000/mm3. On the third day, he deteriorated clinically. His white blood cell count was 20,000/mm3 and his platelet count was 70,000/mm3. The next day, however, his condition further deteriorated and he required inotropes and artificial ventilation. His Hb dropped to 6.4 g%, his white blood cell count increased to 28,000 mm3, and his platelets dropped to 40,000/mm3.

Step 1: Intensive care

- Monitor and stabilize the condition in the intensive care unit. In patients with low platelet count and coagulopathy, insert a catheter into the jugular vein for infusion therapy under ultrasound guidance.

- Refer blood for peripheral blood smear, grouper, cross-match, coagulation, and biochemistry.

Step 2:Assess the severity of thrombocytopenia

- Thrombocytopenia is defined as a platelet count of less than $150 \times 109/L$.

- In critically ill patients, a threshold value of less than $100 \times 109/L$ may be accepted.

- The ability to form a hemostatic clot is maintained as long as the platelet count is at least $100 \times 10 /L^9$

Step 3:Assess the cause of the thrombocytopenia

- A thorough history, physical examination, previous medical records and current usually reveals the cause of the low platelet count.

- Ask about bleeding from other places in the past, such as frequent nosebleeds, bleeding gums, melena, hemoptysis, and blood in stool or urine.

- History of previous platelet counts.

- History of previous blood or platelet transfusions, taking warfarin and antiplatelet agents, including nonsteroidal anti-inflammatory drugs

- Heparin-induced thrombocytopenia (HIT) should be suspected if platelets are reduced by 50% and/or thrombosis occurs 5-14 days after initiation of heparin administration. Assessment of the 4Ts for pretest probability of HIT.

Causes of thrombocytopenia:

- Pseudotrombocytopenia is observed in asymptomatic patients. The presence of platelet clumps in a peripheral blood smear and a normal repeated citrate blood platelet count confirm pseudotrombocytopenia. Automatic counts show thrombocytopenia in some patients due to the presence of giant platelets, but manual platelet counts are normal.

- Diluted thrombocytopenia. Massive blood transfusion.

- Medications (chemotherapy, various drugs), infections - Epstein-Barr virus (VEB), HIV, etc. Infection/Sepsis

- Connective tissue diseases - rheumatoid arthritis, systemic lupus erythematosus, antiphospholipid antibody syndrome.

- Hypersplenism due to portal hypertension.

- Primary bone marrow disease

- HELLP - hemolysis, elevated liver enzymes, low platelet count

- TTP associated with clopidogrel or ticlopidine associated with Gp IIb/IIIa inhibitor -Abciximab

- **Drugs associated with thrombocytopenia:** H2-receptor blockers, drug-dependent antibody (vancomycin, rifampicin, chloroquine, amphotericin B, sulfonamides), Salicylates/NAPs-Aspirin, diclofenac, ibuprofen, Antiepileptic drugs (valproate, carbamazepine, phenytoin), antiarrhythmic drugs (Amiodarone), hapten-dependent antibody (Penicillin, some cephalosporins), Others (quinine, furosemide, thiazide, morphine)

Provocative factors and medications:

Antiarrhythmic agents Procainamide with autoantibody induction mechanism,

Linezolid antibiotics with myelosuppressive effects. Other fluconazole, daptomycin, ganciclovir, nitrofurantoin, piperacillin also provoke thrombocytopenia. Meropenem interaction on folic acid metabolism. Clopidogrel, ticlopidine can cause thrombotic microangiopathy, Unfractionated and low molecular weight heparin. Immune complex with PF4

- Other systemic conditions associated with platelet defects, such as alcoholism, cirrhosis, HIV infection, systemic lupus erythematosus (SLE), and uremia

    - Family history of heavy bleeding.

- Perform a physical examination to look for: signs of bleeding in the skin, mucous membranes, joints, soft tissues, lymphadenopathy, splenomegaly

Step 4: Platelet transfusion

- Three types of platelet products are commonly used in clinical practice: Random Donor Platelets (RDP), Single Donor Platelets (SDP), HLA-compatible platelets

- Platelet transfusion is contraindicated in thrombotic thrombocytopenic purpura (TTP), idiopathic thrombocytopenic purpura (ITP). purpura (ITP) and HIT, unless the patient is bleeding.

Step 5: Evaluate the increase in platelet count after platelet transfusion

- Platelet counts should be measured 10-60 min after transfusion because platelet destruction by the immune system is possible after 10-60 min. Post-transfusion counts after 24 hours assess the survival of platelets that are sensitive to non-immune factors.

- A patient is considered refractory to a platelet transfusion if two or three consecutive transfusions are ineffective.

- Alloimmunization is confirmed by demonstration of antibodies to specifically human leukocyte antigen (HLA) or human platelet antigen (HPA).

Platelet transfusion triggers. Prophylactic blood transfusion in adult patients with a threshold platelet count of 10×10^9 /l. Before placement of a central venous catheter 20×10^9 /l. Urgent diagnostic lumbar puncture 20×10^9 /l, before routine diagnostic lumbar puncture 50×10^9 /l, before major elective surgery (excluding neurosurgery) 50×10^9 /l, in neurosurgery 100×10 /l^9

Factors associated with platelet transfusion refractoriness:

Amphotericin B, vancomycin, ciprofloxacin, heparin;

Patient factors: previous pregnancies, previous transfusions;

Immune factors: HLA, platelet-specific, erythrocyte antibodies;
Duration of platelet *storage;*

Nonimmune *factors*: splenomegaly, fever, infections, bleeding, disseminated intravascular coagulation

Step 6: Understand strategies to improve response to platelet transfusions

- Treat the underlying disease.

- Transfuse platelets identical to the ABO system.

- Transfuse platelets stored for less than 48 hours.

- Increase the number of transfused platelets.

- Choose a compatible donor: HLA-compatible, ABO-compatible.

Step 7: Treat the underlying cause

- Check and discontinue all medications causing the disorder.

- Examine the patient for signs of secondary infection or DIC syndrome.

Initial assessment and cardiopulmonary resuscitation

The management of patients in the ICU who are admitted in a pathologic state is a challenge directly proportional to morbidity and mortality, and a quick and protocol-based ICU regimen will help save these patients.

Step 1: Allocate responsibilities

- Quickly form a team and clearly assign job responsibilities to each member appropriately.

- Initially, the patient should be seen by a senior ICU staff member for initial resuscitation, examination, and management planning.

- Appoint two doctors for initial resuscitation.

- Assign two nurses to unstable patients.

- Seek assistance from other team members in a timely manner if necessary.

Step 2: Begin Initial Assessment and Resuscitation

- The initial goal is to identify immediate life-threatening problems. However, a working diagnosis is necessary to make treatment decisions once physiological stability has been achieved.

- For a patient in cardiac and respiratory arrest, follow the ACLS protocol for
resuscitation to be performed simultaneously, not sequentially, as time is limited.

- For hemodynamically unstable patients, resuscitation should be systematic and focused on assessment and management of A (airway), B (breathing), and C (circulation and consciousness).

- All three components can be monitored simultaneously; a sequential approach is not necessary.

Airway (A).

Assess the airway. The need for definitive airway patency by endotracheal intubation or adjunctive (oral/nasal airway), supraglottic devices, or surgical cricothyroidotomy in patients is based on clinical assessment and should not be delayed.

- Seek help when in doubt about airway obstruction. Look, listen and feel for signs of airway obstruction and secure the airway and intubate if necessary.

Snoring is due to obstruction of the upper airways by the tongue and oropharynx.
soft tissue - introduce the oro/nasopharyngeal airway.

Gurgling - due to upper airway obstruction by secretion - perform aspiration.

Strydor - due to foreign body obstruction or upper airway stenosis, usually on inhalation - remove foreign body or intubate.

Wheezing is due to small airway spasm - give bronchodilators.

Complete airway obstruction *asymptomatic* - intubate.

Respiration (B).

- Assess oxygen demand and ventilation. It can be assessed clinically with pulse oximetry and arterial blood gas analysis:

Look for **clinical signs of respiratory failure**: shortness of breath, tachypnea, inability to speak, breathing with mouth open

Clinical signs of inadequate oxygenation

- Restlessness-Delirium-Drowsiness-Frozen limbs-Cyanosis-Tachycardia-Arrhythmia-Hypotension-Flapping tremor (asterixis).

- The use of auxiliary breathing muscles.

- Paradoxical breathing (abdominal movement inward during breaths) - look for clinical signs indicating inadequate oxygenation or ventilation of the lungs. Remember that these clinical manifestations are a very late sign of respiratory failure and suggest an early cardiorespiratory arrest. Patients should be identified much earlier, and appropriate management should be prescribed.

- Look for signs of tension pneumothorax and signs of massive pleural effusion or hemothorax and drain immediately.

Any signs of massive collapsed lung with desaturation require intubation, suctioning, and positive pressure ventilation.

Some clinical conditions, such as profound loss of consciousness (CCH<8), severe hemodynamic instability, or severe respiratory failure, require immediate endotracheal intubation and mechanical ventilation.

Noninvasive ventilation may be tried in relatively stable patients, for conditions in which noninvasive ventilation can be effective.

- If necessary, use a High Flow oxygen machine.

- Normal oxygen saturation does not preclude impaired airway patency and the need for intubation and pulmonary ventilation.

Circulation (C)

- Assess the adequacy of circulation. Examine the following:

Peripheral and central pulse in frequency, regularity, volume, and symmetry. Skin temperature. Heart rate and rhythm. Arterial pressure (in the supine position and sitting in orthostatic hypotension). Capillary filling. Jugular venous pressure. Diuresis.

Bedside echocardiography - **e-FAST** (enhanced focused ultrasound evaluation for trauma), **RUSH** (rapid ultrasound for shock and hypotension), or **FATE** (this targeted ultrasound examination of heart function for rapid diagnosis or exclusion of various causes of hemodynamic instability, chest pain, acute respiratory failure in critically ill patients)

Consider invasive monitoring - invasive blood pressure, central venous, pressure monitoring including cardiac output. Use volume, inotropes, and vasopressor support judiciously. An early volume test is appropriate in most patients with hypotension. Identify cardiogenic shock and transport to an appropriate institution quickly. Look for pericardial tamponade causing hemodynamic instability requiring immediate pericardiocentesis. Any suspicion of pulmonary thromboembolism should lead to urgent anticoagulant therapy, unless contraindicated, and then take appropriate action. Patients with signs suggestive of aortic dissection should have urgent control of arterial hypertension and heart rate and should be investigated urgently to confirm the diagnosis. In patients with signs of sepsis and septic shock, infusion is used along with rapid administration of broad-spectrum antibiotics.

- Consciousness - Frequent neurologic examination in drowsy patients is necessary. Lateral signs, such as hemiplegia, are usually a sign of neurologic deficit. Decreased consciousness in the absence of a primary neurologic cause is indicative of severe systemic disease. - Check for hypoglycemia and intervene urgently. - Control ongoing seizures with appropriate measures. - Consider urgent antibiotic therapy for patients with signs suggestive of bacterial meningitis.

Exclude *7G*: - Hypovolemia-Hypoxia-Hydrogen ion excess (acidosis)-Hypoglycemia-Hypokalemia-Hyperkalemia-Hypothermia and

5T: - Tension pneumothorax- Cardiac tamponade- Toxins- Thrombosis (pulmonary embolism) - Thrombosis (myocardial infarction). Reversible causes of patient instability can lead to cardiac arrest

Step 3: Focus on the anamnesis.

- Obtain a history from relatives, medical and nursing staff about the unstable patient.

- Review the patient's medical history and perioperative record.

- The presentation of the problem in chronological order with the duration and time profile of the illness should be documented.

- Gather a history of the mechanism of injury in trauma patients.

- Ask about serious comorbidities, such as heart disease, lung disease, kidney disease, previous surgeries, or any other serious health problems in the past.

- Find out about previous hospitalization or use of NIV at home.

- Learn about functional status at home - bedridden, outpatient with support or independent.

- Learn about exercise tolerance.

- In older adults, learn about mental status and cognitive function.

- Gather a detailed history of your medications, including doses and duration of use. Ask about any recent medication changes, allergies to over-the-counter medications, alternative medications, and self-medication.

- Ask about any routine use of sedatives or psychiatric drugs.

- Learn about addictions such as alcohol and tobacco.

- A list of active and inactive problems should be documented in the clinical notes.

- Clarify the resuscitation status of patients at the family's request. Identify next of kin.

Step 4: Do a focused physical exam

- Check vital signs.

- Look for warning signs of serious illness.

- Examine for any life-threatening abnormalities.

Warning signs of severe illness: systolic BP <90 or mean arterial pressure <60 mmHg. , Glasgow Coma Scale score <12, pulse rate >150 or <50 beats/min, respiratory rate >30 or <8/min, and diuresis <0.5 ml/kg/h. CBC, blood sugar, sodium, potassium, urea, creatinine, aspartate aminotransferase (AST), alanine transaminase (ALT), PV, ACTV, arterial blood gases, and lactate levels in sepsis are important for initial evaluation. *Examples of investigations requiring urgent corrective* action-Blood sugar <4 mmol/L or >33 mmol/L-Sodium <110 or >160 mmol/L-Potassium <2.5 or >6.0 mmol/L-PH <7.2 Bicarbonate <16 mmol/L

- Examine for pallor, cyanosis, jaundice, and swelling of the shins.

- Examine your skin for rashes, petechiae, urticariae.

- Systematically examine other organ systems.

- The examination should be repeated frequently for new signs or findings. The Glasgow Coma Scale should be used in neurological patients.

- A chest X-ray and 12-lead ECG should be performed.

- Microbiological cultures must be properly shipped.

- Further investigations should be based on the results of the anamnesis and examination data.

- In unstable patients, investigations should be performed at the patient's bedside as much as possible.

- If transport outside the ICU is required, the patient must be properly supervised and accompanied by qualified personnel

Step 5: recognize a patient at risk

- Take special precautions for the following patient group: The elderly and immunocompromised may not show signs of decompensation, such as fever and tachycardia. In young adult patients, decompensation occurs late because of physiological reserves.

Step 6: Assess response to initial resuscitation

- Assess changes in basic vital signs during initial resuscitation - pulse rate, rhythm, blood pressure, oxygen saturation, diuresis, and mental status.

- Continuous assessment is mandatory.

Step 9: Build a working diagnosis and plan further management

- Initial resuscitation, assessment, examination, and response help make a working diagnosis or provide a basis for a differential diagnosis.
- Re-evaluate the patient frequently to modify the initial plan if necessary.

- Problem-oriented goals and steps to achieve those goals must be identified.

Targeted milestones:

- Mean arterial pressure >65 mmHg. - Continuous invasive blood pressure monitoring - Appropriate infusion therapy - Vasopressor/inotropic support if needed

- Hb > 7 mg/dL, - Monitoring blood Hb levels every 8 hours - Transfusion of red blood cell mass if Hb < 7 g/dL.

- Blood platelet count >10,000 per cc mm- Monitor blood platelet count every 8 hours- Watch for bleeding, if bleeding occurs, transfuse one unit from a single donor (SDP) or 4-6 units of random donor platelets collected from more than one donor (RDP) if SDP is not immediately available.

- RaO2 > 65 mmHg. - Use oxygen masks. - Consider NIVL/invasive ventilation/high nasal flow.
- Adequate and smooth breathing. Provide ventilation support with endotracheal intubation if Glasgow Coma Scale (GCS) < 9, Inhalation of bronchodilators if bronchospasm- Respiratory exercises- Chest physiotherapy- Noninvasive ventilation as indicated.
- Level of consciousness: clear. - Close neurological monitoring - Consider CNS imaging - Consider osmotic therapy
- Diuresis > 30 ml/h- Provide adequate infusion support - Consider renal replacement therapy
- Sedation Assessment = 0-1- Adjust sedation infusion rate according to sedation assessment - Daily interruption of sedation to assess level of consciousness.
- Intra-abdominal pressure (IAP) < 12 mmHg. - Continuous IAP monitoring - Use non-surgical measures to reduce IAP - Consider surgical intervention if medical measures do not help reduce intra-abdominal pressure

Note that this list is not exhaustive.

Step 10: Informing relatives

- After the initial resuscitation, evaluation, and examination, the family should be informed of the likely diagnosis, treatment plan, and approximate prognosis, length of stay, and consent should be taken for any invasive procedures.

Step 11: Documentation and Consent

CHAPTER 5. IMPLICATIONS OF CHEMOTHERAPY AND RADIOTHERAPY FOR ANESTHESIA

Cancer patients are seen by anesthesiologists at various stages of the disease. Anesthesia and surgical intervention for these cancer patients remains challenging because of the challenges associated with the surgical procedure, concomitant cancer therapies such as chemotherapy, radiation therapy, and comorbidities. Therapeutic surgical resection is the primary treatment for potentially curable tumors. Surgery involves the body's stress response, which has metabolic, neuroendocrine, hematologic, and inflammatory/immunologic responses (cytokine stress responses, suppressed cellular immunity. These are major factors in the perioperative immune response and create an environment for possible proliferation of tumor cells leading to metastasis. Other surgical factors include dissemination of tumor cells during surgery. Exposure to pain, blood transfusions, hypothermia, episodes of hypoxia, organ hypoperfusion, hyperglycemia, anesthetic action, and technique on cancer recurrence. These adverse reactions during curative surgical treatment require perioperative intervention by physicians, including anesthesiologists, surgeons, and oncologists, to maintain homeostasis against the effects of both cancer and tissue depletion. Many well-established chemotherapy drugs are antiproliferative agents, targeting rapidly dividing cancer cells, but also damage nonmalignant dividing cells, resulting in toxicity. Chemotherapy usually causes cell death through drug-receptor interactions that stimulate a cascade of catastrophic events, usually leading to apoptosis.

Chemotherapy is broadly classified as: 1. Neoadjuvant chemotherapy : given before surgical resection of the primary tumor, metastases, or both, and designed to shrink the primary tumor. It is also administered to cancer patients at high risk of micrometastatic disease.

2. Adjuvant chemotherapy: prescribed after local treatment (radiation therapy or surgery). Can be used when there are few signs of cancer, but there is a risk of recurrence. Also useful for destroying any cancer cells that have spread to other parts of the body. These micrometastases can be treated with adjuvant chemotherapy, which can reduce the recurrence rates caused by these disseminated cells. After tumor resection to reduce the risk of tumor recurrence.

3. Combination chemotherapy involves treating a patient with a number of different drugs simultaneously. The drugs differ in mechanism of action and side effects. The advantage is to minimize the chances of developing resistance to any one agent. Also, drugs can often be used in lower doses, reducing toxicity. Palliative therapy to improve quality of life and prolong survival without the possibility of treatment.

Combination chemotherapy is often used to increase cancer cell death and decrease drug resistance. The selected drugs may have different mechanisms of action, resulting in a synergistic effect. Chemotherapy is given in "cycles," usually every 2-3 weeks, usually for 3-6 months (but sometimes much longer) with recovery phases between each cycle to restore normal tissue and resolve toxic effects. The use of multi-dose regimens will also increase the likelihood of cancer cell death, since not all cells will be in the susceptible part of the cell cycle with a single injection. Common toxic effects include cardiac, pulmonary, renal, hepatic, gastrointestinal, bone marrow effects, and neurological damage.

Classification of chemotherapeutic agents

Alkylating agents	Antimetabolites	Mitotic inhibitors	Antibiotics	Others

Busulfan	Cytosine	Etoposide	bleomycin	L-asparaginase
Carmustine	arabinoside	Teniposide	dactinomycin	Hydroxyurea
Chlorambucil	Floxuridine	Vinblastine	Daunorubicin	Procarbazine
Cisplatin	Fluorouracil	Vincristine	Doxorubicin	
Cyclophosphamide	Mercaptopurine	Vinidesin	Mitomycin-C	
ifosfamide	Methotrexate	Taxoids	Mitoxantrone	
Melphalan	Pilkamycin			

Mechanism of action of chemotherapeutic agents: 1. blocks the biosynthesis of nucleic acids (DNA, RNA) 2. Directly destroys DNA and inhibits DNA reproduction 3. Prevents transcription and blocks RNA synthesis 4. Prevents protein synthesis and function 5. Affects hormone homeostasis.

Cardiovascular System.

Cardiac toxicity secondary to chemotherapy is common and can be life-threatening. Problems encountered include hypotension, hypertension, arrhythmias, myocardial infarction, congestive heart failure, cardiomyopathy, myocarditis, and pericarditis leading to pericardial effusion and cardiac tamponade. Clinical signs can be acute or late, usually 12 months or more.

Numerous *chemotherapy drugs* cause: 1. Anthracyclines, doxorubicin (adriamycin), daunorubicin and epirubicin are the most common agents involved in developing cardiac toxicity after cancer chemotherapy, but other drugs such as cyclophosphamide, 5-fluorouracil (5-FU), bleomycin, paclitaxel and docetaxel can also cause serious cardiac toxicity. 2. Cyclophosphamide causes direct endothelial damage and hemorrhagic pericarditis or myocarditis. 3. 5ftorouracil was previously thought to cause acute coronary spasm, but recent evidence suggests that this drug also likely causes myocyte toxicity, which is inherently unpredictable except for an increased incidence in patients with a history of coronary heart disease.

Mechanism of Action: The mechanism by which anthracyclines cause cardiac damage is multifactorial, but includes production of free radicals leading to myocyte apoptosis and subsequently to acute and irreversible cardiac damage. Chemotherapeutic drugs tend to damage myocytes. In adulthood, the heart has to functionally adapt to the changes, for example, the ejection fraction may be preserved, but the cardiac reserve is reduced. The damage can be severe and life-threatening. Radiation therapy can be used in conjunction with chemotherapy and can cause damage to heart valves, vessels, and pericardium.

Risk factors for cardiotoxicity include: pre-existing heart disease, concomitant use of chemotherapeutic agents, age at the time of treatment., female gender, current or previous radiation therapy with mediastinal involvement, obesity, LV EF less than 50%.

When evaluating a preoperative patient who has received chemotherapy, we should keep in mind possible cardiac complications. Targeted history taking and examination, it is necessary to look for signs and symptoms of cardiac dysfunction. Of the routine perioperative investigations, an ECG and a two-dimensional echocardiogram should be done. The echocardiogram should focus on specific details of the heart wall, contractility, left ventricular ejection fraction, and pericardial fluid. If necessary, the patient should be referred for evaluation by a cardiologist for optimization prior to surgery. After consultation with the cardiologist, angiotensin-converting enzyme inhibitors should be considered to improve the ejection fraction. The plan of anesthesia during surgery will depend on the preoperative data, the depressant effect of commonly used anesthetics, which may be exacerbated by prior exposure to chemotherapeutic agents even in patients with apparently normal cardiac function. Consequently, all of these patients should be considered at high risk for potential cardiac events during anesthesia and surgery. Invasive monitoring of blood pressure and cardiac output is often required, to maintain normal physiological parameters. Vasopressors should always be on hand to counteract hypotension. ECG alarm limits should be carefully selected to alert the anesthesiologist to any change in electrical activity of the heart. Normothermia should be maintained with a forced air and fluid warming device. This caution should be maintained in the postoperative period as well.

Pulmonary effects:

Cancer patients often suffer from pulmonary complications. 75% to 90% of pulmonary complications are secondary to infection. Pulmonary complications are a serious problem. Respiratory failure in cancer patients who require assisted ventilation is associated with a 75% mortality rate. Pulmonary toxic effects of cytotoxic agents include a combination of direct lung damage and indirect inflammation.

Adverse respiratory effects include:

Early inflammatory interstitial pneumonitis;

Acute noncardiogenic pulmonary edema;

Bronchospasm;

Pleural effusion;

Patients receiving chemotherapy with respiratory symptoms and signs present a diagnostic challenge. Infection, metastatic disease, pulmonary embolism, or drug-induced lesions may be manifestations of possible pulmonary toxicity in a cancer patient.

Drugs commonly causing pulmonary toxicity include:
- Bleomycin-Cyclophosphamide-Nitrourea-Mitomycin-Busulfan-
Methotrexate.

Risk factors for pulmonary toxicity from chemotherapeutic agents include:

- Age older than 70 years- Genetic predisposition- Existing lung disease- History of smoking- Thoracic radiation therapy

The initial manifestation may be subtle, the patient may be asymptomatic without loss of physiologic status or may complain of a dry cough or increased dyspnea with exercise.

There may be minimal changes on chest radiographs and no marker lesions. The pathogenesis of pulmonary toxicity is secondary to chemotherapy.

Methotrexate and *cyclophosphan* classically cause pneumonitis. Treatment is often unsuccessful and progressive pulmonary fibrosis may develop.

Because of the immunosuppressive effects of chemotherapeutic drugs (most chemotherapeutic agents cause myelosuppression, including neutropenia), patients may experience acute malaise with infections such as pneumonia. These patients may require a period of artificial respiration in the postoperative period.

Bleomycin is a particularly important chemotherapeutic drug that the anesthesiologist should be aware of. Bleomycin is often used to treat germ cell tumors and Hodgkin's disease can progress to life-threatening pulmonary fibrosis. Pulmonary toxicity occurs in 6-10% of patients and can be fatal.

Pneumonitis develops gradually in the first few months of treatment, but may persist for up to 6 months of treatment. Pneumonitis is accompanied by increased fibroblast activity. Fibroblast activity is followed by collagen synthesis and decreased collagen degradation, resulting in pulmonary fibrosis. Exposure to highly concentrated oxygen therapy, even for short periods of time during anesthesia often causes rapidly progressive pulmonary toxicity in patients previously treated with bleomycin. These claims have been considered controversial, but it is recommended that any patient previously treated with bleomycin be treated as a high-risk patient.

The bleomycin-induced lung damage usually occurs unnoticed within the first 6 months of starting treatment, but the possibility that high inhaled oxygen fractions will provoke pulmonary toxicity remains a lifelong risk. All patients who have ever received bleomycin should have a warning card and a warning label placed in their records. Symptoms of bleomycin-induced pulmonary toxicity are nonspecific and include dry cough and shortness of breath. Patients may also experience pleuritic chest pain and fever. On examination, pulmonary rales and hypoxemia may be found. The diagnosis of bleomycin toxicity should be considered for all respiratory illnesses in patients who have ever received bleomycin.

Bleomycin toxicity has typical manifestations *radiologically:*

- Linear interstitial shadows may be seen, which may be similar to the Curley B lines seen in pulmonary edema.

- A confluent airspace shadow may be present, which could be diagnosed as an infection if the diagnosis of bleomycin lung lesions is not considered.

- Pneumothorax and pneumomediastinum are well-recognized complications of severe bleomycin-induced lung damage.

Of particular concern are patients who have undergone surgery and undergone bleomycin treatment. Oxygen therapy can both induce and exacerbate bleomycin-induced lung damage.

Hyperoxia is the delivery of inhaled oxygen at a concentration equal to or greater than 30%. The concentration of inhaled oxygen increases the risk of developing bleomycin-induced lung damage, while lower inhaled oxygen concentrations decrease the risk. When bleomycin was preoperative, lower oxygen concentrations should be used during anesthesia and postoperatively. Preoperative evaluation of a patient with prior exposure to bleomycin will require a careful history taking. Depending on clinical findings, necessary investigations may include chest radiographs, arterial blood gas analysis, computed tomography of the lungs, pulmonary function tests, and bronchoscopy. Oxygen should be prescribed in the medication chart, and the oxygen dose should be adjusted frequently to maintain a minimum exposure to achieve a target peripheral oxygen saturation range of 88% to 92%. If oxygen saturation is higher than this, oxygen should be discontinued or the dose reduced. Ventilation strategies involving the use of PEEP and careful fluid balance will limit the amount of oxygen needed.

In the postoperative period, chest physiotherapy, a good anesthetic regimen, and early mobilization will also minimize the need for oxygen.

Renal system.

Some chemotherapy drugs are nephrotoxic and cause acute or chronic renal failure. These patients subsequently have a higher incidence of arterial hypertension leading to cardiovascular disease. Acute renal failure may develop within 24 hours after administration of a single dose of cisplatin. Adequate hydration with forced diuresis appears to reduce the incidence of renal toxicity. The use of saline is particularly useful because high concentrations of chloride in the tubules inhibit hydrolysis of cisplatin. Renal toxicity may increase if the patient receives aminoglycosides at the same time. Newer cisplatin analogues such as carboplatin and oxaloplatin are less nephrotoxic with equal efficacy against malignancies.

- Ifosfamide can cause proximal tubule abnormalities.

- Cyclophosphamide can cause hemorrhagic cystitis

- Mitomycin C is associated with a syndrome involving

microangiopathic hemolytic anemia and renal failure. Of particular importance to the anesthesiologist is the knowledge that the nephrotoxic process is exacerbated by dehydration and concomitant administration of nonsteroidal anti-inflammatory drugs.

Careful fluid optimization and administration of analgesics are mandatory in the perioperative period.

Nervous System.

Chemotherapy can damage any part of the human nervous system. The most common agents with neurotoxic side effects important to the anesthesiologist are vincristine and cisplatin. The periwinkle alkaloid ***vincristine*** can cause serious neurotoxicity. It can be used to treat lymphoma and leukemia. Vincristine can cause peripheral neuropathy, muscle pain, cranial neuropathy, and seizures. Of particular concern are the effects on the autonomic nervous system with the development of orthostatic hypotension and the rare but serious condition of vocal cord paralysis. Vincristine may also aggravate preexisting neurological conditions.

- ***Methotrexate*** in high doses is used to treat, among other cancers, bone cancer, sarcoma, and can cause acute encephalopathy, including confusion, seizures, hemiparesis, and coma (usually reversible).

- ***Ifosfamide*** also classically causes encephalopathy, especially in women with large pelvic tumors.

- ***Paclitaxel*** and oxaloplatin usually cause peripheral neuropathy with the effects of chemotherapy. The onset is acute, occurring within 12 to 24 hours of treatment. Nausea and vomiting occur 24 hours later and may last 6 to 7 days.

- ***Cisplatin*** in high doses causes nausea and vomiting within 24 hours in 90% of patients not taking prophylactic anti-emetics. Patients with vomiting are at risk for electrolyte imbalances, dehydration, weight loss and malnutrition. Preventing aspiration remains the primary concern of anesthesiologists and anesthesiologists, and this patient population is at increased risk. A complete neurological exam should be performed before surgery and documented to identify any neurological damage. MSU researcher Geoffroy Laumet and his team and an interdisciplinary team of scientists from the University of Lille, University of Strasbourg and Pasteur Institute in Lille in France and the University of Coimbra in Portugal found that isradefylline, a drug already FDA-approved and used to treat Parkinson's disease, can reduce the side effects of cisplatin while maintaining its anticancer power. **https://msutoday.msu.edu.**

- Regional anesthesia is relatively contraindicated in any patient with neurologic side effects after chemotherapy treatment and it is appropriate to document deficits before anesthesia.

Gastrointestinal system

Gastrointestinal toxicity often occurs after the administration of most chemotherapy drugs. The effects of chemotherapy occur on rapidly dividing cells throughout the gastrointestinal tract and there is potentially significant mucosal damage throughout the tract. Gastrointestinal toxicity includes nausea, vomiting, mucositis, and diarrhea. Chemotherapy regimens containing *5-FU* and *irinotecan* have been associated with a significantly higher risk of chemotherapy-induced diarrhea. Not surprisingly, dehydration can occur. In these cases, the water-electrolyte balance is compromised and must be corrected before surgical intervention is indicated. In patients with severe nausea and vomiting, rapid sequential induction of anesthesia to prevent aspiration should be considered. Direct trauma due to laryngoscopy will exacerbate mucositis caused by chemotherapy and may cause severe bleeding, leading to difficulty visualizing the airway.

Liver system.

Disorders of liver function such as cirrhosis and clotting disorders are frequent consequences of cancer chemotherapy. Abnormal liver function tests are a common problem in cancer patients with possible causes including liver metastases, infections, liver disease (e.g., alcoholic liver disease), and hepatotoxic medications. Chemotherapy-related liver damage may also occur, including parenchymal damage with fatty changes, cholestasis, and hepatocellular necrosis. ***Methotrexate*** is known to cause cirrhosis and liver fibrosis.   Diffuse hepatocellular destruction has been seen secondary to ***cyclophosphamide*** treatment. Many chemotherapeutic drugs are metabolized in the liver and, as such, require dose reduction if liver function is impaired.

Metabolism in the liver must be considered, and isoflurane is the preferred volatile agent. Halothane should be avoided. Vecuronium and rocuronium should be used with caution and closely monitored. The usual precautions for dosing anesthetics in patients with liver disease should be used, and regional anesthesia may be contraindicated because of associated coagulopathy.

The hematopoietic system.

Most chemotherapy drugs affect bone marrow and peripheral blood cells, resulting in myelosuppression. Life-threatening sepsis and rapid deterioration can occur if a patient develops an infection with neutropenia. Symptoms and signs may be atypical; fever may be absent.

Appropriate broad-spectrum antibiotics should be administered immediately. Pancytopenia can have serious implications for anesthesia and surgery, causing decreased oxygen-carrying capacity, increased risk of bleeding, and opportunistic infection. Bone marrow function should be carefully evaluated before anesthesia. Consultation with a hematologist should be considered. Myelosuppression is usually partial or completely reversible within 6 weeks of cessation of chemotherapy, but in some patients may be longer-term.

Various side effects of chemotherapeutic agents. Steroid use.

The cancer patient often has a history of exogenous administration of glucocorticoids as part of a chemotherapy regimen. A patient who has received ≥ 2 weeks of
glucocorticoids within the past year is considered at risk for depressed adrenal function. However, many of these patients are capable of a normal stress response.

Chemotherapy and wound healing

The outcome of surgical interventions may be affected by impaired wound healing caused by the antitumor drugs used to treat the underlying tumor. Neutropenia that accompanies some chemotherapy for 7-10 days after administration can affect the early phases of wound healing. Most patients with leukocyte counts of $500/mm^3$ have no side effects of leukopenia on surgical wound healing. Chronic anemia also has little effect on surgical wound healing. The effects of chemotherapy directly on wound healing depend on the dose and timing of drug administration. A high incidence of wound complications has been reported in women undergoing mastectomy after preoperative chemotherapy and radiation therapy.

Tumor lysis syndrome

In extremely large tumors and cancers with a high white blood cell count, such as lymphomas, teratomas, and some leukemias, some patients develop tumor lysis syndrome with rapid destruction of cancer cells causing the release of intracellular contents into the blood. High levels of uric acid, potassium, and phosphate are detected in the blood. High phosphate levels cause secondary hypoparathyroidism, which leads to lower blood calcium levels. This causes kidney damage, and high potassium levels can cause cardiac arrhythmias. Although prophylaxis is available and often done in patients with large tumors, it is a dangerous side effect that can lead to death if left untreated.

Radiation therapy is when radiation is delivered to a specific area of the body to try to cure cancer. The purpose of the radiation is to destroy rapidly dividing cancer cells while sparing the slower dividing somatic cells. Radiation is usually used in conjunction with surgery or chemotherapy, making it difficult to separate the effects resulting from each of these treatments. Radiation can be delivered by a machine outside the body (distant radiation therapy) or it can come from radioactive material placed inside the body (internal radiation therapy, also called brachytherapy). The type of radiation used depends on: - Type of cancer - Size

- Location - How close the tumor is to normal tissue - How far the radiation beam should travel - General health and medical history - Other treatments - Age and other conditions

External radiation therapy

Most often delivered as photon beams (X-rays or gamma rays). Three-dimensional conformal radiation therapy (3D-CRT): The most common type. Intensity Modulated Radiation Therapy (IMRT)

- The dosage is adjusted for different areas of the tumor and surrounding tissue

- Powerful computer program calculates the required number of beams and angles

- Goal: Increase dose in areas that need it and reduce exposure to sensitive areas

- May reduce the risk of some side effects

- A larger volume of normal tissue is irradiated as a whole. Image-Guided Radiation Therapy (IGRT)

- Multiple image scans during treatment.

- Can improve accuracy and allow for a reduction in planned treatment volume
- Reducing the total radiation dose to normal tissues. Tomotherapy
- IMRT type under visual control
- Hybrid between a CT scan and a remote radiation therapy unit
- Protection of normal tissues from high doses of radiation

Stereotactic radiosurgery

- Can deliver one or more high doses of radiation to a small tumor.

- Extremely precise targeting and positioning of the tumor under visual control

- A high dose of radiation can be delivered without excessive damage to normal tissue.

- Radiation therapy in fewer sessions

- Smaller radiation fields are used

- Treat tumors outside the brain and spinal cord- Usually administer more than one dose

- Can only treat small, isolated tumors; including lung and liver cancer.

Proton therapy

- Gives up most of its energy at the end of its path (Bragg's peak) and gives up less energy in passing with reduced exposure to normal tissue.

Internal radiation therapy (brachytherapy):

Interstitial: uses a radiation source placed inside tumor tissue.

Intracavitary: Uses a source placed in a surgical or body cavity.

Systemic radiation therapy

Ingested or receives an injection of a radioactive substance or radioactive substance bound to a monoclonal antibody.

Examples: radioactive iodine, ibritumomabtiuxetan (Zevalin), combined tositumomab and iodine I 131 tositumomab (Bexar), samarium-

153-lexidronam (Quadramet) and strontium-89 chloride (Metastron).

Side effects

Depends on body area treated, dose administered per day, total dose, general medical condition, and other treatments.

Acute (early)

- Skin irritation - Damage to exposed areas (salivary glands or hair loss in head or neck treatment) - Problems with urination (lower abdominal treatment) - Fatigue - Nausea with or without vomiting

- Most disappear after treatment ends (some may be permanent)

Chronic (late onset)

- May or may not occur

- Fibrosis (replacement of normal tissue with scar tissue) - Bowel damage - Memory loss - Infertility - Second cancer (rare); highest in those treated for cancer in childhood or adolescence.

Systemic effects: 1. Gastrointestinal tract.

Radiation *esophagitis*: often involved in radiation therapy for lung cancer, especially when using chemosensitizers. Symptoms usually disappear 1-3 weeks after irradiation. Symptoms: impaired peristalsis, odynophagia (pain when swallowing) and dysphagia.

Radiation *enterocolitis*: often leads to fibrosis leading to intestinal strictures, obstruction, fistulas with abscess formation, ulceration with bleeding and malabsorption.

Acute radiation *enteritis* - reduced absorption surface area leading to decreased absorption of nutrients and possible dehydration and malnutrition. Symptoms: diarrhea, abdominal cramps, and nausea. Chronic radiation enteritis - symptoms do not appear for 6 months to 25 years after treatment and usually require more serious treatment. Other symptoms may include dry mouth, anorexia, and stomatitis (inflammation of the mouth).

2. Pulmonary

Radiation-induced lung disease.

Radiation pneumonitis (acute): interstitial inflammation leading to a decrease in the amount of oxygen involved in lung metabolism. This can occur 1-6 months after radiation exposure and usually goes away in 6-12 years.

months.

Symptoms: dry cough with shortness of breath on exercise or may change to a severe cough with shortness of breath at rest.

Radiation *fibrosis* (chronic): progressive and occurs several months after radiation therapy. Other problems may include bronchopleural fistulas, pneumothorax, hemoptysis, and bronchial asthma.

3. Cardiovascular

Radiation heart disease - can lead to pericarditis, coronary heart disease, myocardial disease and aortic valve disease

4. Musculoskeletal System.

Connective tissue involvement- late changes such as fibrosis, atrophy are common, especially in collagen- In the bones and limbs it can cause weakness, limb length discrepancy and scoliosis- It can cause edema and decreased range of motion- It can cause pelvic adhesions that lead to painful movements and sometimes plexopathy- Lymphatic system it can cause loss of flexibility by vascular contractility.

Although true lymph vessels can retain their shape, fibrosis in the surrounding tissue can inhibit vascular growth in the tissue that needs to be healed.

5. Nervous System.

Acute symptoms: occur during treatment and include debilitating fatigue; may result in short-term memory loss, changes in behavior and cognition, decreased appetite, dry skin, hearing loss, hair loss, and reduced salivation. Subacute symptoms: occur 1-4 months after treatment and are less common. Radiation to the cervical spine may lead to subacute myelopathy (Lhermitte's symptom). Brainstem radiation can lead to ataxia, nystagmus, and dysarthria. Chronic symptoms: occur months or years after therapy and may include brain damage, vascular damage that leads to ischemic heart disease, transient ischemic attacks, stroke, or myocardial infarction.

Radionecrosis is the result of whole brain radiation therapy. Secondary tumors may develop and the hypothalamic system may be affected. Symptoms: headache, changes in consciousness and personality, focal neurological disorders and seizures.

Myelopathy - occurs as a result of exposure of the spinal cord. May present as Brown-Sequard syndrome or motor neuron syndrome.

Plexopathy - occurs as a result of damage to the brachial and lumbar plexuses. Symptoms may include paresthesias, motor deficits, lymphedema, and pain.

6. Skin

Radiation dermatitis - common because it is used in most cases of radiation therapy.

7. Miscellaneous:

Lymphedema.

- Risk factors: Axillary surgery/radiation therapy. Volume of local surgery. Local radiation exposure. Delayed wound healing. Tumor causing lymphatic obstruction.

Radiation Fibrosis Syndrome. Progressive fibrotic sclerosis of tissue as a result of radiation therapy. It affects many different types of tissue, including skin, muscle, ligaments, tendons, nerves, heart, lung, gastrointestinal, genitourinary tract, and bone; for a structure to be considered affected by this syndrome, it must be within the radiation field or have tendon, neurovascular innervation or lymphatic flow passing through that area.

The interaction between the anesthesiologist and the cancer patient begins with a preoperative visit for surgery.

The purposes of such a preoperative visit may be as follows:

1. to optimize the physical condition of the patient.

2. To assess the impact of cancer and cancer treatments (chemotherapy, radiation therapy, and surgery) on the patient.

The role of the anesthesiologist in the preoperative examination and preparation of the surgical patient has intraoperative and postoperative management. This begins with a thorough anamnesis and physical examination. It should be individualized according to comorbidities such as chronic obstructive pulmonary disease (COPD), bronchitis, arterial hypertension, coronary heart disease and diabetes mellitus. The choice of perioperative treatment should be based not only on age, but also on the general condition of the patient.

Preoperative evaluation should include a history of smoking, alcohol abuse, and respiratory problems.
Respiratory, respiratory, cardiovascular, renal, neurological, and hepatic systems need careful evaluation.

Anesthesiologists should gather an appropriate history related to prior surgery and anesthesia, as this may affect postoperative management.

Investigations:

Routine clinical tests such as - CBC, - Urinalysis, - Serum electrolytes, - Blood sugar levels, - LFT - RFT - BUN, S. creatinine - Pulmonary function tests, - Arterial blood gas analysis, - Chest x-ray and ECG. - ECHO was included in all patients who received chemotherapy to assess LV function and regional wall motion abnormalities, and to obtain other cardiac-related information.

Past cancer treatment (surgery, radiation therapy, chemotherapy) can affect anesthesia management. Chemotherapy is often used to enhance the response of cancer cells to radiation therapy, but can have adverse effects depending on the specific agents used, the cumulative dose, and the toxicity of the drug. The most common are pulmonary and cardiac toxicity. Commonly used chemotherapy agents are cisplatin, fluorouracil, methotrexate, carboplatin, and paclitaxel. Methotrexate, paclitaxel, and docetaxel cause myelosuppression, leading to thrombocytopenia and neutropenia. Paclitaxel and carboplatin can cause a decrease of more than 20% in carbon monoxide diffusivity, which may persist for five months after completion of chemotherapy. Reckzen et al. described interstitial pneumonia in patients receiving paclitaxel in combination with radiation therapy because of lymphocytopenia. Gastrointestinal toxicity leading to oral mucositis, diarrhea, weight loss, and electrolyte imbalances can occur with methotrexate. Cisplatin and docetaxel can cause central nervous systemic damage.

Heart problems:

Chemotherapeutic agents can cause impaired cardiac contractility, arrhythmias (anthracycline antibiotics), cardiomyopathy (anthracycline), myocardial tissue damage (cyclophosphamide), endocardial fibrosis (busulfan) and QT interval prolongation (doxorubicin). Clinical manifestations include pericarditis, congestive heart failure, ischemic chest pain and arrhythmia syndromes. The ECG may show decreased QRS complex voltages, the systolic time interval may be increased, and the ejection fraction as well as fractional shortening may be decreased. Congestive heart failure is treated with diuretics, glycosides and oxygen. Huttman and colleagues have shown that previous anthracycline treatment can increase the depressing effects of anesthetics even in individuals with healthy cardiac function at rest.

Radiation therapy causes dose-dependent endocardial and myocardial fibrosis, which can lead to restrictive cardiomyopathy. The anesthesiologist should be aware that various cancer therapies can cause pathology in patients with normal hearts or exacerbate pre-existing cardiac problems.

Operating room and postoperative monitoring should include ECG, diuresis, central venous pressure, and, when possible, pulmonary artery pressure and occlusion pressure in selected patients.

Pulmonary problems:

Cancer patients may have treatment-induced lung damage, which can manifest as noncardiogenic pulmonary edema, chronic pneumonitis, and fibrosis. Because these patients have a weakened immune system, they are more prone to secondary infection, often affecting the lungs.

Pneumonitis and pulmonary fibrosis can be caused by many chemotherapeutic agents.

A history or symptoms suggestive of shortness of breath with exercise or shortness of breath at rest should alert the physician. Arterial blood gases are required in addition to chest radiographs. Pulmonary function tests, including arterial blood gases, spirometry, and diffusion capacity should be evaluated. Findings compatible with interstitial fibrosis include: increased alveolar-arterial gradient, restrictive lung disease, and decreased diffusing capacity. Patients receiving bleomycin therapy should not receive high doses of oxygen concentration and restrictive infusion should be preferred both during and after surgery. Ventilation support should be expected in the postoperative period.

Other problems:

Immunosuppression occurs with all alkylating agents. Close attention must be paid to asepsis in the perioperative period. In cancer patients metabolic disorders caused by tumor factors or tumor destruction by antitumor therapy may develop. Tumor lysis syndrome is a known complication associated with cancer. Thus, serum electrolytes should be included in the study panel. Common sites of cancer metastasis are the liver, lungs, brain, spine, and bones. These can cause location-specific symptoms, so systemic evaluation should include these locations as well.

Hepatotoxicity can occur with most anticancer drugs. Busulfan, methotrexate,
cisplatinum, and others, which may cause nephrotoxicity, should not be administered.

Nutritional status and preoperative nutrition is another problem. Several authors have reported malnutrition in most cancer patients and especially in head and neck cancer patients with compromised airways. Balanced electrolyte solutions taken the evening before surgery will help maintain optimal renal blood flow and glomerular filtration.

Potentially nephrotoxic drugs should be avoided. The effects of cyclophosphamide, a pseudocholinesterase inhibitor, may persist for 3-4 weeks after their use, and there is a recognized risk due to interaction of the drug with suxamethonium (a depolarizing myorelaxant metabolized by pseudocholinesterase), causing a risk of prolonged postoperative apnea. Toxicity to the central and autonomic nervous system and the occurrence of peripheral neuropathies can occur with vincristine, cisplatin, and others. Therefore, regional anesthesia is also contraindicated. Preoperative sensory conditions and neurologic deficits should be documented. The anticholinesterase effects of alkylating agents are significant. Reduced dosage of succinylcholine is indicated to prevent prolonged respiratory depression.

Inhibition of monoamine oxidase may occur with the administration of procarbazine. Because of the synergistic effects of barbiturates, antihistamines, phenothiazines, narcotics, and tricyclic antidepressants and they should be used with caution. Diarrhea is a side effect of many anticancer drugs. Serum electrolytes and volemic abnormalities should be corrected preoperatively as well as in the postoperative period. Patients may have elevated levels of anxiety and nervousness prior to surgery and appropriate premedication should be recommended. Excessive sedation should be avoided during premedication in elderly patients, especially those with head and neck lesions with anticipated airway obstruction.

Airway problems: Airway problems are of paramount importance in patients with head and neck cancer. They often present difficulties in the operating room that make mask ventilation and tracheal intubation difficult. There are certain preoperative indicators that help predict potential airway obstruction, such as voice changes, history of dyspnea, dysphagia, exercise intolerance, head and neck irradiation and prior head and neck surgery, perianesthesia, breathing and tumor obstruction, and swelling of the larynx and pharynx. A history of difficulty breathing while lying down but not on the side or stomach may indicate a mass in the pharynx, neck, or anterior mediastinum. Pain relief for such a patient may result in severe airway obstruction. People with stridor should have a laryngoscopy and bronchoscopy to evaluate the airway. A coarse, hoarse voice indicates a vocal cleft tumor; a muffled voice indicates a supraglottic tumor. History of snoring and sleep apnea may indicate the presence of a tumor mass. Information should be gathered about the duration, probable cause in the position that exacerbates the stridor. The presence of wheezing, cyanosis, chest retraction, and bloating of the nose should also be considered.

Radiation therapy often results in restriction of jaw movements, stiffness of the fixed cervical spine due to the development of radiation fibrosis. In addition, the larynx and trachea may become resistant to external finger pressure manipulation during tracheal intubation. Thus, tracheal intubation may be difficult. Careful physical examination of the tissues, especially between the submandibular and hyoid regions, may indicate potential obstruction of airway patency. The submandibular space in these patients may be affected due to post-radiation fibrosis. In some patients, the larynx may appear anterior in spite of a normal submandibular distance due to fibrosed submandibular space. Radiation therapy may also obliterate the lymph vessels, resulting in increased postoperative edema. Patients may experience acute side effects of radiation therapy in the form of an inflammatory reaction that results in epidermitis and oral mucositis and are prone to infection and bleeding during airway manipulation. Patients who have undergone surgical resections of tumors may have an easy airway, but the same patient when coming in for reoperation may cause difficulty in airway patency because of distorted airway anatomy.

Radiologic studies to assess airway status in patients with head and neck cancer, which can be relatively asymptomatic, can help in predicting difficult intubation. CT can also provide insight into tracheal compression, if present. Clear communication between the surgeon and anesthesiologist is important for proper perioperative management of the patient and it should always be remembered that cancer surgery is urgent.

Airway management

For head and neck cancer, it is best to proceed with conscious fiberoptic intubation under sedation. Indirect laryngoscopy can provide the anesthesiologist with much useful information, such as airway anatomy, location of the tumor. Damage to the 9, 10, 12 cranial nerves from tumor invasion or due to surgical resection may predispose the patient to aspiration or obstruction. Inhalational induction while maintaining spontaneous ventilation rather than intravenous induction with myorelaxants is a safe option. Nasal intubation is usually preferred for maxillofacial surgery. Various techniques such as fibrobronchoscopy-guided intubation, transtracheal jet ventilation, retrograde tracheal intubation, and tracheostomy should be well known to anesthesiologists working with cancer patients.

Positioning

Major oncologic surgeries are time-consuming. In view of the long operation, the patient's positioning with soft pressure point padding. In such surgeries, the arms are usually turned to the patient's side, insulated, and care must be taken to prevent compression of vascular and nerve structures.

Monitoring

In addition to routine monitoring, invasive monitoring such as arterial pressure and venous pressure monitoring may be required, major surgery with anticipated blood loss or due to disease. Arterial cannulas should be placed for major surgery with expected blood loss and hemodynamic monitoring. Arterial cannulas should not be placed in the same arm if a radial forearm flap is planned. Two large-diameter cannulas or central vein catheterization should be for major surgery. Bladder catheterization and temperature control are necessary.

Intraoperative airway management

Intraoperative airway problems such as kinked, disconnected endotracheal tube can occur in patients undergoing head and neck surgery because of the proximity of the airway to the surgical field. Airway monitoring should include capnography, peak inspiratory pressure, and breath sounds. The endotracheal tube and connectors should not be kinked and should be securely attached. Whenever possible, the breathing circuit attached to the endotracheal tube should be secured to the patient's head to allow the surgeon to reposition the head if necessary without causing accidental extubation. Care should be taken at all times to ensure that the breathing circuit does not pull the breathing circuit downward.

Maintaining anesthesia

It is important to maintain body temperature during surgery. Intraoperative hypothermia should be avoided. Various methods are used to maintain body temperature, such as warming and humidifying inspiratory gases, a forced-air warming blanket, and warm intravenous fluids. At the end of surgery, the oropharyngeal swab, if used in head and neck surgeries, should be removed and the oropharynx sanitized. If there is postoperative edema involving structures that could potentially block the airway, the patient should be closely monitored and possibly extubation should be delayed. Extubation may be attempted after the patient is fully awake and there are no signs of ongoing bleeding and edema.

Extubation

Patients who have undergone extensive surgery with massive blood loss and hemodynamic instability may require continued postoperative ventilatory support. In any neck or head surgery and in which a tracheostomy is not established, the timing of extubation is critical. This will depend on various factors, such as the degree of edema and the resulting upper airway deformity. In a patient who has undergone prolonged surgery, including free flap reconstruction, the trachea may remain intubated and the patient may be sedated overnight in the ICU. Other patients may be extubated in the operating room or post-operative ICU when they are fully conscious. Airway patency equipment at the beginning of anesthesia should always be on hand and available also during extubation. Airway swelling and surgical changes in the anatomy may prevent adequate mask ventilation if acute airway obstruction develops after extubation.

Pain management in cancer

Pain can be directly related to cancer progression or to therapies to treat cancer. When a patient with cancer-related pain enters the operating room, anesthesiologists need to know what type of pain the patient is experiencing and how much and what medications the patient is taking. Patients with moderate to severe pain syndromes controlled with oral opioids may have a high tolerance for drugs and benzodiazepines. Patients with severe pain associated with cancer who require parenteral drug administration with or without adjuvant are very difficult to treat in the operating room. It is critical that these patients remain on their analgesics. The patient may have narcotic withdrawal during surgery (hypertension, tachycardia, and sweating). Additional narcotics are administered as needed during surgery. Epidural anesthesia may be considered in patients undergoing thoracic, abdominal, and lower extremity surgery.

The impact of anesthesia on cancer surgery. (https://resources.wfsahq.org/atotw/implications-of-anaesthesia-on-cancer-surgery)

The perioperative period is characterized by physiological stress, which can affect tumor cell survival. The response to surgical stress, the inflammatory response, the effects of anesthesia techniques and anesthesia pharmacological agents are all factors that contribute to a state of relative immunosuppression in the perioperative period. Immunosuppressed patients often have high levels of catecholamines, growth factors, and prostaglandins, which can stimulate metastatic transition of cancer cells. Local tissue damage during surgery causes inflammation that promotes the release of cytokines such as interleukin-6 and prostaglandin E, which typically inhibit the activity of natural killer cells, which typically play an

important role in the detection and destruction of circulating cancer cells during surgery. Multiple perioperative factors can lead to a state of decreased perfusion and localized hypoxia. Hypoxia leads to an increase in hypoxia-inducible factor-1-a (HIF1a) and vascular endothelial growth factor. HIF1a promotes tissue repair and cell proliferation in damaged cells, but can
unintentionally affect the metastasis of cancer cells. Vascular endothelial growth factor promotes angiogenesis and lymphatic vessel dilation, allowing cancer cells to spread through the vascular and lymphatic systems.

Total intravenous anesthesia versus volatile anesthetics

Recent studies show that the inhalational anesthesia method can have a negative effect on patients with cancer, while the total intravenous anesthesia (TIVA) can be helpful.

Inhaled agents increase tumor growth factors, such as HIF1.and insulin-like growth factor, which promote tumor cell growth, invasion, and migration. In contrast, propofol appears to reduce HIF1.a levels and exhibit antioxidant and anti-inflammatory properties, making TIVA preferable for maintenance anesthesia in cancer surgery. Unfortunately, data on the clinical outcomes of propofol-based TIVA compared with volatile anesthetics are limited to retrospective cohort studies. To date, there have been no prospective randomized controlled trials (RCTs) comparing TIVA and inhaled anesthesia in cancer outcomes; however, some are in development.

Regional Anesthesia. Over the past 20 years, there have been conflicting studies on the effects of regional anesthesia on cancer outcomes. Regional anesthesia has several theoretical advantages with regard to cancer recurrence. These include pain control and the ability to minimize opioid consumption due to immunosuppression, decreased stress response to surgery, and the direct immunomodulatory effect of local anesthetics. Several randomized controlled trials have not shown any benefit of regional anesthesia in terms of cancer recurrence or survival. A large RCT by Sessler et al. studied the effects of regional anesthesia on breast cancer patients. More than 2,100 patients were randomized to receive regional anesthesia (paravertebral block and propofol sedation) or inhalational anesthesia with opioid-based analgesia. The RCT showed no significant differences between the two groups with regard to cancer recurrence. Another RCT Du et al. analyzed patients who underwent extensive surgery for abdominal or thoracic cancer and could not show an improvement in cancer recurrence or survival in patients who received a combined epidural and general anesthesia technique compared with general anesthesia alone.

Lidocaine (lidocaine). Local anesthetics can alter cancer outcomes as a direct result of their immunomodulatory receptor suppression effect epithelial growth factor, interleukin-1, tumor necrosis factor alpha, and nuclear factor kappa B. can reduce the stress response to surgery and attenuate the associated immunosuppression. The literature is unclear, with conflicting data regarding overall survival and recurrence-free survival. Lidocaine reduces cell migration and cancer viability in laboratory studies. Retrospective cohort studies suggest that intraoperative intravenous lidocaine administration is associated with improved cancer outcomes; however, further studies in this area are needed to provide clarity.

Blood transfusion. Cancer surgery can cause significant blood loss requiring blood transfusions. Laboratory studies have proven that blood transfusion causes inflammation and immunosuppression, which may subsequently contribute to cancer recurrence. Clinical studies suggest that perioperative blood transfusion in cancer surgery can have a deleterious effect on outcomes. A 2006 Cochrane review that included 12,000 patients concluded that blood transfusion was associated with a risk of colorectal cancer recurrence (odds ratio 1.42; 95% confidence interval 1.20 to 1.67). Other meta-analyses have confirmed a significant recurrence rate associated with bladder, stomach, and prostate cancer. On the other hand, data on blood transfusion are currently limited to meta-analyses involving retrospective studies in which an association, but not necessarily causality, can be established.

Opioids. Opioid analgesia is commonly used for perioperative pain management in cancer patients, but recent trends and advances in accelerated recovery programs have encouraged a shift toward a multimodal approach to pain management. Opioids could theoretically affect tumor growth and metastasis through a number of mechanisms. They have immunosuppressive properties, including the reduction of activity of natural killer cells and neutrophils, which can accelerate cancer progression. Opioids can directly affect cancer cell growth in vitro by acting on the mu-opioid receptor, which is overexpressed in a wide range of cancer cells, including breast, colon, and lung cancer cells. Clinical research in this area is limited and cannot provide conclusive evidence of the deleterious effects of perioperative opioid use in cancer patients. Despite the paucity of data in this area, it is clear that a balance must be sought between the competing effects of reducing the stress response associated with opioids and cancer progression.

In general, it seems reasonable to practice an opioid-saving technique whenever possible.

Alpha-2 agonists. Alpha-2 adrenoreceptors are known to disrupt norepinephrine release to attenuate the sympathetic stress response; however, to date, there are few data on the effects of alpha-2 agonists on immune system modulation and cancer recurrence. Alpha-2 receptor agonists (e.g., dexmedetomidine and clonidine) have been increasingly used in recent years for sedation and opioid-sparing analgesia. Laboratory studies mostly indicate increased tumor growth and metastasis of alpha-2 agonists and mostly harmful effects on cancer cell lines. Nevertheless, the potential tumor-enhancing effects of alpha-2 agonists need to be balanced with secondary opioids and inhaled drugs in cancer surgery.

Steroids. Steroids have known immunosuppressive properties. It follows that they may affect the immune system's ability to detect and destroy circulating tumor cells and potentially increase the risk of tumor recurrence. Steroids also have anti-inflammatory properties that may lessen the surgical stress response and the negative effects associated with it. Steroids are commonly used in the perioperative setting as anti-emetics, anti-inflammatories, and analgesics. Studies examining the clinical outcomes of steroid use in the perioperative period are limited to retrospective cohort studies and yield mixed results, with most showing no difference in survival or recurrence rates. Higher-quality randomized trials are needed to establish the benefits or risks of steroid use in patients with perioperative cancer. Current data on steroid use in oncologic surgery are insufficient to recommend a change in current clinical practice in this area.

Nonsteroidal anti-inflammatory drugs

An inflammatory response to surgery is associated with cancer recurrence, so anti-inflammatory drugs could theoretically reverse this effect. Potential beneficial effects of nonsteroidal anti-inflammatory drugs include opioid-saving effects, altered expression of epithelial growth factor receptor and nuclear factor kappa-B, and inhibition of prostaglandin-induced immunosuppression. Despite the theoretical benefits of nonsteroidal anti-inflammatory drugs, clinical perioperative studies after cancer surgery are inconclusive.

Return to assigned cancer treatment (RIOT).

RIOT is a new endpoint in oncologic surgical trials. Reduced surgical recovery time allows for earlier RIOT, thereby increasing the likelihood of recurrence-free survival. Postoperative complications, usually related to anesthesia techniques, can reduce or prolong a patient's recovery, which may require resumption of oncologic therapy. Hayden et al. conducted an RCT examining the effect of intraperitoneal ropivacaine infiltration on readiness for postoperative oncologic therapy. They found a reduction in time to RIOT with ropivacaine infiltration compared with controls. This was the first RCT on oncoanesthesia using RIOT as the primary endpoint. Although the use of RIOT as an endpoint in oncoanesthesia studies to date is limited, it could be a potentially useful endpoint in the future.

Recommended reading

1. Buddeberg BS, Seeberger MD. Anesthesia and oncology: friend or foe? Front Oncol. 2022;12:802210.

2. Sherwin A, Wall T, Buggy DJ. Anaesthesia and cancer recurrence: UpToDate; 2022. Accessed June 28, 2022. https://www.uptodate.com/contents/anesthesia-and-cancer-recurrence#H2875951382.

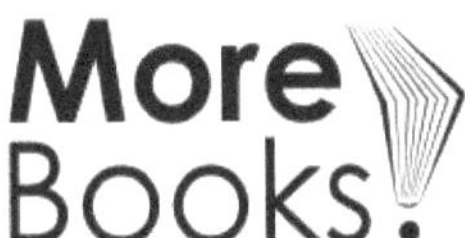

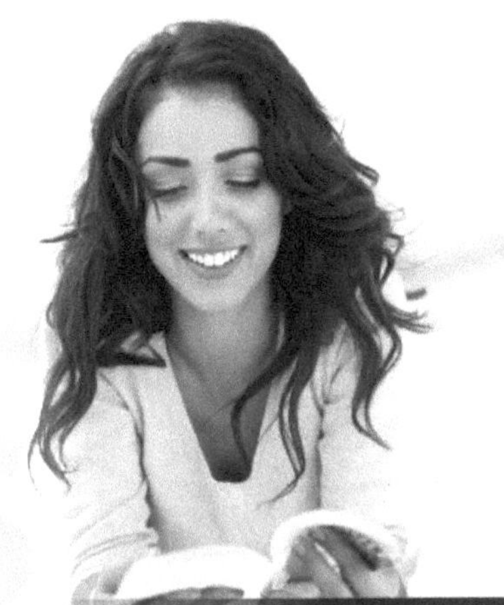

I want morebooks!

Buy your books fast and straightforward online - at one of world's fastest growing online book stores! Environmentally sound due to Print-on-Demand technologies.

Buy your books online at
www.morebooks.shop

Kaufen Sie Ihre Bücher schnell und unkompliziert online – auf einer der am schnellsten wachsenden Buchhandelsplattformen weltweit! Dank Print-On-Demand umwelt- und ressourcenschonend produziert.

Bücher schneller online kaufen
www.morebooks.shop

info@omniscriptum.com
www.omniscriptum.com

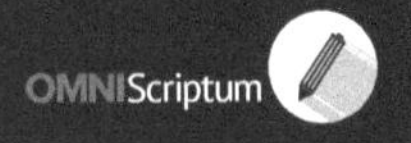

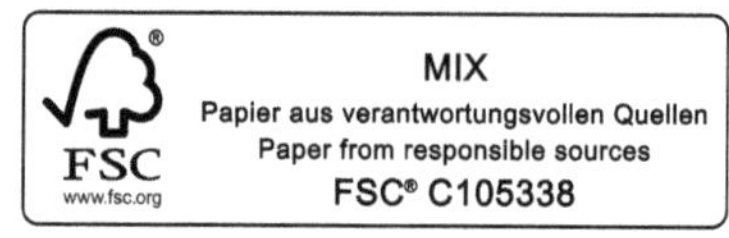
FSC
www.fsc.org
MIX
Papier aus verantwortungsvollen Quellen
Paper from responsible sources
FSC® C105338